THE
HEALTH
PRACTICE
MANAGEMENT
Handbook

EDITED BY
DAVID
LOSHAK

**KOGAN
PAGE**

First edition published in 1992

This edition (second) in 1993

Apart from any fair dealing for the purposes of research or
private study, or criticism or review, as permitted under the
Copyright, Designs and Patents Act, 1988, this publication may
only be reproduced, stored or transmitted, in any form, or by
any means, with the prior permission in writing of the
publishers, or in the case of reprographic reproduction in
accordance with the terms of licences issued by the Copyright
Licencing Agency. Enquiries concerning reproduction outside
those terms should be sent to the publishers at the
undermentioned address:

Kogan Page Ltd
120 Pentonville Road
London N1 9JN

© Kogan Page 1993 and © Medical Defence Union (Chapter 1.5)

British Library Cataloguing in Publication Data

A CIP record for this book is available from the British Library.

ISBN 0 7494 0982 7

ISSN 1351 4679

Typeset by DP Photosetting, Aylesbury, Bucks
Printed and bound in England by Clays Ltd, St Ives plc.

THE
HEALTH
PRACTICE
MANAGEMENT
Handbook

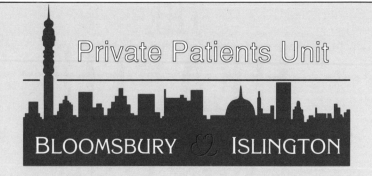

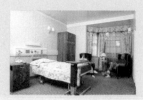 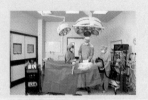

Contents

Foreword *Virginia Bottomley JP MP, Secretary of State for Health*   **9**

Introduction *David Loshak*   **11**

The Contributors   **13**

PART ONE: BUSINESS PLANNING

1.1   **The Role of the Practice Manager**   **17**
      Mo Rillands

1.2   **Strategic Planning in General Practice**   **24**
      Eric Finlayson

1.3   **Communications Systems in General Medical Practice**   **30**
      Michael Hamilton

1.4   **Drawing up a Business Plan**   **40**
      Kathie Applebee

1.5   **The Legal Aspects of Health Practice Management**   **47**
      Angela Cullen

PART TWO: HUMAN RESOURCE MANAGEMENT

2.1   **Managing People**   **57**
      Merrill Whalen

2.2   **Building a Practice Team**   **69**
      Susie Lawson

2.3 Training   76
Trevor Illsley

PART THREE: FINANCIAL PLANNING

3.1 Organising Practice Finances   83
John Dean

3.2 Controlling Practice Finances   93
John Dean

3.3 GP Fundholding   102
Jackie Roberts

3.4 Taxation and the GP   109
Angela Britton

PART FOUR: PATIENT CARE

4.1 Community Nursing Services   117
Lynn Young

4.2 Prescribing and Formulary   125
Dr David Clegg

4.3 Nursing and Residential Homes   131
Pauline Ford

4.4 New Health and Safety Regulations   137
Norman Ellis

PART FIVE: MANAGING PREMISES AND EQUIPMENT

5.1 Premises, Equipment and Maintenance   149
Angela Scott

5.2 Choosing a Laboratory   168
David Browning

5.3 Health and Safety in the Surgery   175
Norman Ellis

Contents

5.4 Looking to the Future   184
       Sally Irvine

**PART SIX: DIRECTORY OF PRODUCTS, SERVICES AND
SUPPLIERS TO THE HEALTH CARE INDUSTRY**

6.1 Directory of Products, Services and Suppliers to the Health
       Care Industry   193

6.2 Useful Addresses   219

Index of Advertisers   223

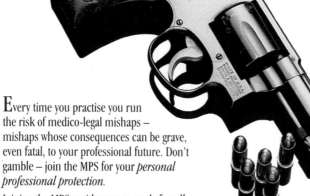
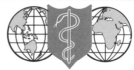

Foreword

General practice is the front door to the National Health Service. For many people it is their only point of contact with health care professionals. Good quality primary care is the backbone of the modern NHS and will play an increasingly important role as we move towards the 21st century.

A high standard of care for the patient is inseparable from the effective use of the money available for it. The NHS will always face increasing demands on finite resources. Quality management initiatives, which combine improved services with better efficiency, are an important way of addressing the problem. At the same time, we must be careful not to turn health care into a factory experience, where patients feel that they are being 'processed' through a system. The quality of care for the individual is as important as the quantity of patients treated.

The recent changes in the NHS have given GPs and other health professionals working in primary care a much stronger voice. The return to local decision-making has been widely welcomed. The reforms have provided a framework with which we are better able to identify patients' needs and respond to them. Professional staff and managers are developing a better understanding of their respective roles, leading to more effective working and improved care for patients.

This patient-centred approach to quality is very much part of the *Patient's Charter*. Many family health service authorities, individual doctors and primary health teams have taken enormous strides forward to improve the delivery of services to their patients. The development of the primary care charter will help level up standards in primary care to those of the best.

The introduction of the fundholding scheme has combined the two great skills of the family doctor – that of medical expertise and the small business. The role of the practice manager will become increasingly important to GPs empowered with the resources they need to buy services for their patients.

As I visit individual practices and clinics around the country, I am constantly impressed by the energy and enthusiasm which managers and staff are bringing to their work. I welcome the timely publication of this Handbook and commend you in your continuing drive to raise standards in practice management.

Virginia Bottomley JP MP
Secretary of State for Health

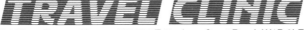
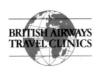
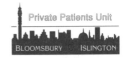

Introduction

The practice manager has rightly been described in a *British Medical Journal* editorial as 'a rising star' in general practice. One could fairly say 'the' rising star.

The recent television resurrection of Dr Finlay and his casebook will doubtless have tweaked many a nostalgic nerve, but nostalgia was largely what it was. The days when the doctor's dutiful wife took calls and made appointments for her husband, probably a single-handed practitioner whose surgery was in the front room at home, are, if not entirely over, certainly and rapidly on the way out, for a host of social, economic, political, medical and technological reasons. General practice has changed radically. It has become 'primary health care', a far wider concept involving many professionals besides the GP. The group practice of the 1990s is a multi-disciplinary enterprise providing a range of services which go well beyond straightforward diagnosis and empirical treatment into such areas as health promotion, ill-health prevention, social work, nursing, patient advocacy, rehabilitation, resource allocation and community relations.

Running a practice therefore needs professional management for which the doctor, whose own tasks require far wider medical knowledge and involve far more complex considerations than in the past, has neither the time nor expertise. It demands training and skills which require a professionalism in its own right. The modern group practice without a practice manager would be a plane without a pilot.

At first, as group practices began to grow in numbers and responsibilities, senior receptionists took on the job, but they were little more than *ad hoc* administrators at that stage. It soon became clear that the modern group practice must not merely be run, but managed, managed in order to cope with constant and often drastic change, growing responsibilities, rising patient expectations and expanding need. The practice manager must plan and organise and delegate, run a tight ship, ensure compliance with an array of laws and regulations, and take responsibility for matters ranging from overall finance to everyday housekeeping.

'Under the new contract, there will be winners and losers among general practitioners', says the *British Medical Journal*. 'Those with a good practice manager will more likely find themselves among the winners'. It is the aim of this Handbook to help them be so.

David Loshak

The Contributors

Kathie Applebee is a management and training consultant with Practice Consultancy Services, Swindon.

Virginia Bottomley has been Secretary of State for Health since April, 1992.

Angela Britton is a partner with chartered accountants Touche Ross & Co, specialising in personal and partnership taxation.

David Browning is Manager of Birmingham Pathology Services, the trading name of South Birmingham Health Authority Pathology Services.

Dr David Clegg is Medical Adviser to Wolverhampton Primary Health Care Unit and Family Health Services Authority.

Angela Cullen is a former practice manager who is Practice Manager Adviser of the Medical Defence Union.

John Dean is an accountant based in Surrey who specialises in general practice finance.

Normal Ellis is Head of the General Practice Division of the British Medical Association, London.

Eric Finlayson is a Management Consultant with Salford University Business Services Ltd.

Pauline Ford is a Royal College of Nursing Adviser in Policy and Practice developments as they affect nursing and older people.

Michael Hamilton handles professional communications services at the Scottish Software Partner Centre, South Queensferry, Scotland.

Trevor Illsley is training facilitator for Practice 2000.

Sally Irvine is General Administrator of the Royal College of General

Physicians and provides management consultancy to GPs and practice managers.

Susie Lawson has been a practice manager in Morpeth, Northumberland, for the past 11 years.

David Loshak is a freelance writer and journalist specialising in health, medicine and science.

Mo Rillands is Chief Executive of a general practice in Gosforth.

Jackie Roberts is an independent consultant accountant specialising in the financial training of fundholding practices and manages the Department of Health funded Manual of Accounts helpline for fundholding practices.

Angela Scott is practice manager of a six-partner group general practice in Leighton Buzzard.

Merrill Whalen is Head of Training at AMI Ross Hall Hospital, Glasgow.

Lynn Young is Community Health Adviser at the Royal College of Nursing, London.

Part One

Business Planning

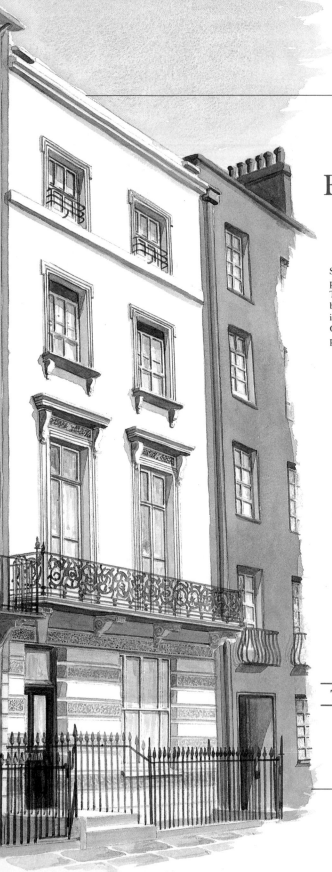

THE ENDOCRINE CENTRE

Situated in the heart of the world's premier location for private medicine The Endocrine Centre is rapidly becoming a major centre for research into treatments for the Menopause and Osteoporosis. The Endocrine Centre provides:

◊

Full Clinical and Gynaecological examinations by Consultants in Gynaecology and Endocrinology

◊

Haematological and Histological screening

◊

Bone Mineral Density Scanning for Osteoporosis

◊

Individual Consultations and Comparative Clinical Studies to full G.C.P. standards

◊

For further details of our services please contact:

THE ADMINISTRATOR
THE ENDOCRINE CENTRE
69 WIMPOLE STREET
LONDON W1M 7DE

Telephone 071 935 2440
Telefax 071 224 6649

THE ENDOCRINE CENTRE

The Role of the Practice Manager

Mo Rillands

Introduction

Since 1948, when the NHS came into being, general practice (primary health care) has been the funnel through which 95 per cent of all patients pass before being referred to hospital and/or social services. However, during this time it remained largely untouched by NHS re-organisation; although a management revolution occurred in the hospital service, management in general practice was patchy and performed largely by staff with no formal management training or qualifications.

In 1990, the Government introduced major reforms to the NHS (NHS & Community Care Act, 1990). This changed the focus and direction of primary health care, with more emphasis on the management of disease prevention and health promotion. There is now a clearer division of roles and responsibilities, with services being provided to meet contracts which specify the services required, including performance, quality and cost. Moreover, the Patient's Charter stresses the importance of service users. For the first time, services are to be provided and met to clearly defined national and local standards, in ways responsive to people's views and needs. Furthermore, the views of consumers, and assessment of their health and care needs, are now acknowledged as central to the approach of management in planning and delivering services.

The culture change

The purchaser–provider split and the 1990 GP contract revolutionised general practice not only in terms of accountability for the services

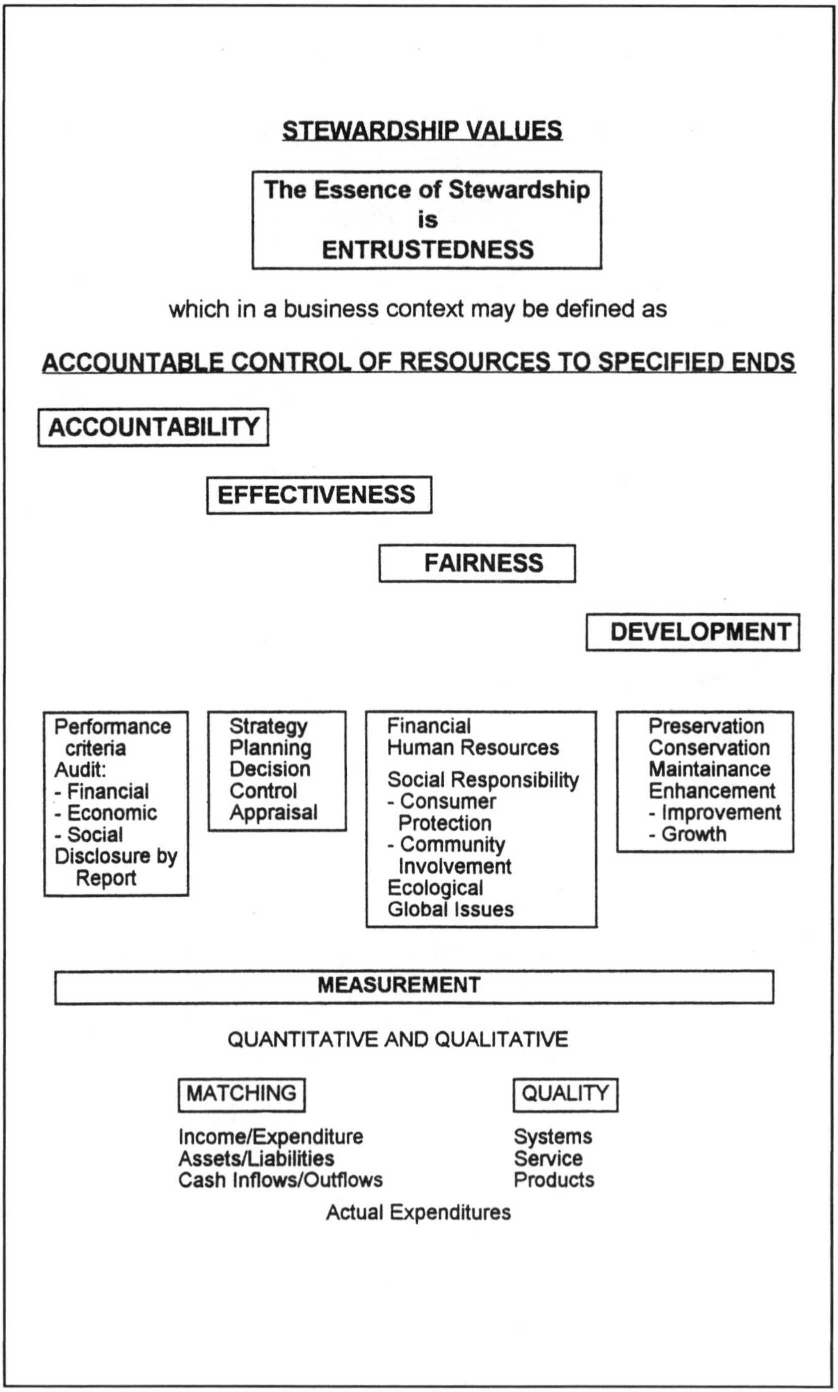

STEWARDSHIP VALUES

**The Essence of Stewardship
is
ENTRUSTEDNESS**

which in a business context may be defined as

ACCOUNTABLE CONTROL OF RESOURCES TO SPECIFIED ENDS

ACCOUNTABILITY

EFFECTIVENESS

FAIRNESS

DEVELOPMENT

Performance criteria Audit: - Financial - Economic - Social Disclosure by Report	Strategy Planning Decision Control Appraisal	Financial Human Resources Social Responsibility - Consumer Protection - Community Involvement Ecological Global Issues	Preservation Conservation Maintainance Enhancement - Improvement - Growth

MEASUREMENT

QUANTITATIVE AND QUALITATIVE

MATCHING   **QUALITY**

Income/Expenditure   Systems
Assets/Liabilities   Service
Cash Inflows/Outflows   Products

Actual Expenditures

Figure 1.1.1 *Stewardship values*

provided, but also in the managerial expertise necessary to deliver services which meet both targets and service specification.

The requirements for business planning, cash flow forecasts and clinical financial audit, the need to market services and to meet the demands of the Patient's Charter, and the management of staff, are all part of the revolution in general practice. They signal a cultural change from the traditional stand-alone practice to the concept of the primary health care team as a managed team and a business. The practice administrator role is no longer appropriate in a market-orientated environment that needs general management expertise to succeed.

Achieving cultural change

It is the role of the practice manager to manage strategic change. However, it is unrealistic to suppose that this can be implemented if current beliefs, assumptions and ways of doing of things remain the same. Today's manager needs leadership and co-ordinator qualities together with well-honed interpersonal skills to facilitate delivery of effective health care and health gain from a multi-disciplinary team.

The practice manager's major aim should be to enable and empower the primary health care team to deliver the full range of services appropriate to the practice population.

Stewardship values

Management in general practice today can perhaps be best described as 'stewardship' which in a business context may be defined as accountable control of resources (financial and human) to meet specified ends – health care gain.

The practice manager is entrusted to use and manage resources efficiently to secure the objectives of the practice. This includes the values of the partners, patients and staff. The Patient's Charter has raised expectations and encouraged general practice to accept that services should be customer rather than producer driven. Consumerism has enhanced the patients' role and makes them major stakeholders in the business. Similarly, the introduction of managers from the NHS and industry, together with information technology and finance staff, has made general practice staff key stakeholders in the business too.

It is the role of the practice manager to manage the interests of the

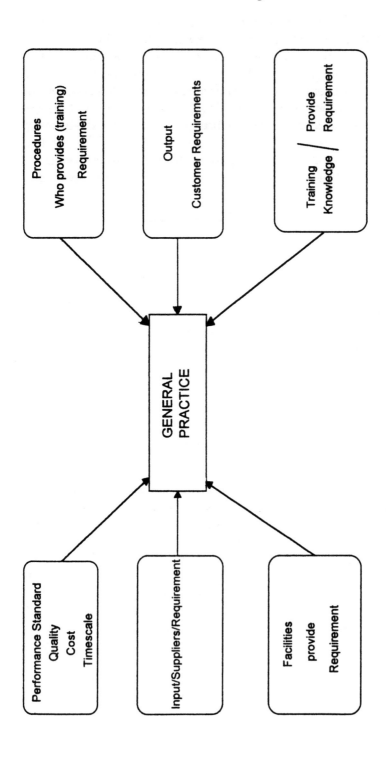

QUALITY MANAGEMENT

Procedures
Who provides (training)
Requirement

Output
Customer Requirements

Training / Provide
Knowledge / Requirement

GENERAL
PRACTICE

Performance Standard
Quality
Cost
Timescale

Input/Suppliers/Requirement

Facilities
provide
Requirement

Figure 1.1.2 *Quality management*

authentic stakeholders in a way that allows equity of access to services for patients and a harmonious working environment for staff. However, it is inevitable that some priorities will depend upon both economic and ethical considerations, and this will inevitably lead to tensions.

The stewardship model for practice management, and the idea that ethics and taking account of authentic stakeholders pays, is useful, but covers only some of the issues in business and health care. However, the model is useful in handling values in general practice systematically because it addresses both the stewardship (entrustedness) and the company (the GPs') values, while allowing the practice manager to take account of the environment (legislation, health and safety, equal opportunities).

Accountability

The practice manager is accountable to the partners for the system's operational management of performance criteria in relation to income and expenditure and cash inflows, outflows, and expenditure. Certainly, monies from targets are dependent on both quantitative and qualitative data being available to show that both quality and the appropriate quantity have been achieved (with smears, for instance).

Effectiveness

A clear and systematic approach to business planning is central to the success of any business and the aims and objectives of the practice should be known to all the staff. National data, demographic practice information and trends, health indices, sources of funding, hospital and community resources and quality of care (complaints, re-admissions), should be used by the practice manager to plan services. Outcomes of care and usage rates should be compared and used to prepare a purchasing strategy.

Fairness

The people who work in general practice are its greatest resource and the practice manager's role should be to enable and empower the primary health care team to deliver the full range of planned services to the practice population. This should include working and forging links with all relevant agencies to provide the best in seamless primary health care.

Staff should be encouraged to give a quality, consumer-orientated service through training and team building so that value for money is obtained for the services required. However, appropriate levels of pay, conditions and pensions should be used to promote goodwill and promote equity in the primary health care team. Accessibility and availability of the services provided should be promoted and marketed by the practice manager. Lack of uptake of any service should be targeted to protect the 'stakeholders' (patients) to promote consumerism and future public health targets.

Development

Nothing in life is certain so it is inevitable that changes in technology and drugs will affect and possibly improve plans for delivering health care, as with key hole surgery or drugs for the treatment of benign prostatic hyperplasia instead of prostactectomy. Therefore, strategies and purchasing plans need to be reviewed, monitored and updated. As more procedures are done in the community of general practice, the development of premises and the skilling of staff will develop.

Technology, with the benefits for better patient care in terms of disease index, morbidity and mortality data and soft data to assist in needs assessment, will need to be seen as a growth and development area.

Summary

The practice manager of today is both a leader and a generalist, able to use and interpret information technology data, able to read a balance sheet, forecast cash flows, and comfortable with sensitivity ('what if') analysis. Able to motivate and enable the primary health care team and to engender trust from the partners, today's practice manager is a strategist who takes account of external issues such as finite resources and EC legislation, while balancing this with internal ethics in relation to delivering value for money health care.

Quality management is the umbrella that the modern practice manager uses to bring the jigsaw that is general practice together. It provides a role model that understands the competition of the market, knows that quality brings cost benefits and job satisfaction, and helps to deliver the best use of resources. However, the culture of the NHS and general practice, and the lack of security together with the complexity of case management where many disciplines are involved, mean that ideology and lack of communication can disable or even destroy the best laid plans. Above all, today's practice manager is a good communicator – health gain can only be achieved if every piece of the jigsaw is in its place all the time.

The practice manager is not only the organiser and co-ordinator of this jigsaw called general practice, but the master planner.

1.2

Strategic Planning in General Practice

Eric Finlayson

The NHS annual reporting cycle obliges GP fundholding practices and those in the final run-up to fundholding to prepare business plans. While these notionally help the funding agencies to prepare their budgets, the process by which they are produced often makes them of little real value, least of all to the practices themselves.

When Salford University Business Services decided to combine its experience in health care management with that of developing business plans in the private sector, it found an extraordinarily complex situation. The general practitioner is, in effect, managing three or four businesses, each with its own demands:

- the clinical management of patients' health and well-being;

- running a financially viable business partnership;

- satisfying the bureaucratic demands of the paper-driven NHS machine;

- managing the fund on behalf of the NHS.

Together, these produce an exceptionally demanding management task, if the business and its strategic direction are to be controlled. Family health service authorities are too new to have established an effective framework for supporting practices in this way, so many practices have to look elsewhere for experience and advice on consolidating the business and building for the future.

Some have already discovered the Government's *Enterprise Initiative*. This develops businesses through subsidised management consultancy in a range of specialisations, including business planning,

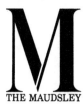
marketing, financial and management information systems, operational processes and systems, and quality.

This scheme offers practices:

- careful selection of those consultancies and their consultants qualified to provide this assistance;

- free help from the Department of Trade and Industry (DTI) to assess the needs of the clients and to negotiate with consultants;

- quality assurance of every consultancy job delivered under the initiative;

- negotiated 'bulk' consultancy fee rates;

- a grant which pays up to half the cost of the consultancy.

To take advantage of this grant, a practice has only to contact a listed consultancy firm. My organisation will advise a practice free of charge about the scheme and help with the grant application.

The purpose of the strategic business plan in general practice is to help the partners to develop a blueprint for the future of the practice by:

- examining all aspects of the practice, its community, and environment;

- clearly establishing what the partners want to achieve;

- identifying and evaluating the strategic options;

- mapping out a firm action plan to implement the strategy.

Since completing its first strategic planning exercises for general practitioners and dentists more than a year ago, Salford University Business Services has worked with many practices, learning by stages and perfecting an approach which brings in a full range of issues under the partners' control. These include:

- clinical and non-clinical objectives;

- market position;

- staffing structure, responsibilities, and training;

- patient satisfaction and quality of service;

- the use of information and information technology;

- practice finances;

- planning and controlling the effective use of the fund.

The business plan must set out the strategic objectives of the practice, both clinical and non-clinical, based on the aspirations and interests of the partners. With the partners, the consultant examines the internal strengths and weaknesses of the practice. The market position of the practice is set out with respect to its community, socio-economic environment and trends, and with other practices in the locality.

The importance of people in the practice must be given due consideration. That means reviewing the organisation's structure, skill mix and capabilities, the interests of the partners and staff, their jobs and relationships, and their training needs.

Quality and patient satisfaction are of growing importance as expectations become more sophisticated. The consultant will usually conduct a patient satisfaction survey during the first half of the planning process. He will then feed the results into decision-making and the choice of priorities. Broad quality issues in the practice are addressed through developing an understanding of needs and expectations, processes, and the culture of the practice.

Information is essential for developing the practice as a business and in raising clinical achievement. A strategy for exploiting what the practice has, how it will extend this to support its outstanding objectives, and priorities and time scales need to be set out for discussion and agreement.

The process involves recognising where the practice is, where it wants to get to, and how it will get there, by identifying the range of strategic options, such as whether to expand, develop services, rent, buy, develop the partnership, and work to achieve new targets. These options are evaluated, particularly in terms of workload and their financial impact. The partners can then agree the strategy and, as a final stage, produce a detailed action plan. Without this clear, committed planning, the strategic plan remains a mere intellectual exercise.

While most, though not all, such assignments are carried out under the 'business planning' umbrella of the *Enterprise Initiative*, we clearly have to combine the full range of management consultancy skills, bringing in quality, marketing, information systems, human resource development, health care, health economics, and even design when options are being explored in depth.

When we first tried to make sense of practice finances and to relate financial achievement to activity and clinical achievement, we came up against the Red Book. It is difficult to think of any other sphere of business which is regulated by 260 pages of fine print, rules and figures. The only effective and efficient solution was to use computers to produce a program which would allow us to input details of practice size, shape, and achievements and to model the financial outcomes, right down to the profit shares due to individual partners. Of course, this meant building in all significant parts of the Red Book, to avoid the need for looking up the rules and figures and carrying out arithmetic calculations.

The strategic planning tool we produced allows our consultants to work alongside the practice and to provide instant answers to the 'what if' questions in considering all the options. The real outcomes of choices often differ greatly from guesses based on experience and intuition, even if forecast only over just one year, rather than the five years which the *Strategic Planner* predicts.

A strategic plan must be treated as a live, working document and remain a blueprint for the future. As circumstances, environments and people change, therefore, the plan must also evolve. The *Strategic*

Planner has been built as a consultant's tool but, as the skills of strategic planning are transferred to general practitioners and their practice staff, they too must be able to use the computer system. Sponsorship by a major pharmaceutical company has allowed Salford University Business Services to redevelop the *Strategy 2000 GP Strategic Planner* as a robust and fully packaged end-user product. It is now available to any practice which wants to try its hand at forecasting its results, and to exploit informed decision-making in developing and maintaining practice strategy.

The long-term partnership set up under this sponsorship and distribution agreement will ensure that the *Strategic Planner* is updated to match developments in the Red Book. It will be extended to new areas of decision-support in GP practice and fundholding, based on the lessons constantly being learned by working alongside general practitioners and by identifying new and common problems and their solutions.

For those who need help in developing the strategic and management skills they need to thrive in today's climate of rapid change, there are various packages of consultancy assistance. The DTI's *Enterprise Initiative* scheme is open until 31 March 1994. Consultancy grants for practices will then cease, but the consultancy service will continue for those general practitioners who see it as a cost-effective use of a small part of their management allowance.

The benefits of strategic planning are best judged by practices themselves. Those identified by the partners and staff involved are:

- reduction in partners' administrative workload;

- control of the future of the practice;

- elimination of guesswork from business decisions;

- improved planning and direction for developing services;

- maximising business surpluses;

- greater efficiency, effectiveness and quality;

- more effective use of information and information technology.

Feeling that they are too busy, many practices are still deferring essential strategic planning exercises. But all practices are hard-pressed, and things will not get any easier until they make the effort to step back a pace and develop strategies to increase:

- quality of service;

- profitability;
- job satisfaction.

By putting off strategic planning, the future for a general practice will only remain uncertain.

Communications Systems in General Medical Practice

Michael Hamilton

Introduction

This chapter will examine the theory and practice of communications systems in general medical practice, and suggests an action plan to make sure that communications in the practice are up to standard. It also looks at aspects of new communications technology and offers some hints on confidentiality.

In general practice, poor communication can cause complaints, legal actions and, as anyone who attends inquests and fatal accident inquiries knows, can also be a contributory factor in avoidable deaths. The regular audit and improvement of communications in medical practice is therefore no luxury but essential.

Communication defined

A good definition of communication for our purposes is 'the transfer of information and ideas from one person or system to another'.

Information and ideas are transferred to others not only in writing and speech but in the form of data, tables, diagrams and graphs.

Ideally:

- the sender will express his or her information or ideas in a language or other format which cannot be misunderstood or misinterpreted;

- there will be perfect transmission by speech or other medium;

- at the end of the communication process, the sender and the recipient will have an exact understanding of each other.

Good communication results when the meaning of speech or data, tables, graphs or diagrams, is accurately and unambiguously expressed, transmitted, received and interpreted without error.

Communication between people

But in practice, people do not always express their ideas or information clearly. Nor do they always use an appropriate medium. There are often inherent defects in the chosen communication system or its capacity.

As a result, communications problems that arise include messages that are misunderstood, messages that must be sent again and again before they are received (the engaged fax number!), messages that are not transmitted at all or received by the wrong recipient, and messages that arrive at the destination but are not received by the addressee.

Three imperatives

There are three main imperatives for communication in general medical practice:

- CLARITY: the sender must make the information or ideas, and the addressee, unmistakably clear;

- EFFICIENCY: the communications medium must be efficient;

- CONFIDENTIALITY: information must be sent only to authorised recipients and no-one must be overheard.

An action plan

Before seeking to improve communications in the practice, practice managers should identify existing problems and prepare an action plan suitable for their size of practice. It is essential that the doctors agree to it. Practice managers should:

- find out the perceived communication problems of the practice;

- start with a written questionnaire;

- follow it up with interviews;

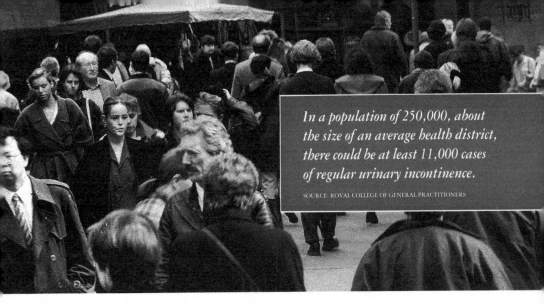

In a population of 250,000, about the size of an average health district, there could be at least 11,000 cases of regular urinary incontinence.

SOURCE: ROYAL COLLEGE OF GENERAL PRACTITIONERS

Faces in a crowd.
But which one has the incontinence problem?

Although over 3 million people in the United Kingdom suffer from incontinence, thanks to the Aquadry range from DePuy Healthcare their problem need not be obvious.

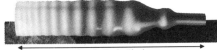

Aquadry Freedom Sheath

The Aquadry range of quality incontinence products has several components. Aquadry Freedom, and the shorter length Freedom Plus sheaths are the only true one-piece sheaths with no liners or applicators and so will give both security and convenience for patients and carers alike.

Aquadry Leg Bags have a contoured shape which is designed to fit the leg closely, and superior leg straps, fabric backing and a secure lever ▶ tap. Aquadry leg bags are available in a range of capacities.

Short inlet tubes, or long-adjustable inlet tubes are available on all bags.

◀ The final link in the Aquadry system are the Aquadry 2 litre drainage bags for overnight use.

All these products are available on prescription.

You might expect to pay a premium for this level of quality but one look at your tariff will tell you otherwise!

If you would like to receive a *free* Starter Pack of Aquadry

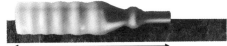

Aquadry Freedom Plus shorter length sheath

products to try with your patients, all you have to do is return the FREEPOST coupon, today.

FREE STARTER PACK!

AQUADRY. THE *RIGHT* CONTINENCE CARE AT THE *RIGHT* PRICE!

SERVICES TO PRACTICE MANAGERS FROM DEPUTY HEALTHCARE

1. Thackraycare – continence and stoma appliance services, offering specialist nursing advice and prescription dispensing and delivery.

With so much more emphasis being placed on to providing the best possible care in the community you may find that there are simply not enough hours in the day to fulfill the needs; Thackraycare may be able to help you.

Thackraycare work with members of the practice team and alongside continence professionals to offer advice, expert fitting and follow up support to patients requiring incontinence or ostomy appliances. Based around care centres thoughout the UK our highly skilled team of appliance nurse specialists provide the highest standards of care. With their experience in, and access to, all appliances available on Drug Tariff, their fitting takes into account both the needs of the patient and the most cost effective prescribing for the practice.

For further information on how Thackraycare can help you to more cost effective prescribing of ostomy and incontinence products or simply some advice in this field contact Elaine Westerman Customer Relations Officer free on 0800 526177.

2. Practice Plus – an efficient and expert mail order service for the cost conscious practice. The leading brands and the latest products in diagnostic equipment and a range of cost effective infection control products for General Practice. Practice Plus assures you of the best attention at all times; both with customer service and after sales support in the form of comprehensive warranties and with our efficient nationwide delivery.

From the simplicity of a tendon hammer to the sophistication of the electrocardiogram Practice Plus can help; choose from the catalogue, then telephone or post your order and your choice will be delivered to you within 48 hours if stock is available.

For more information a copy of our catalogue and details of our single order discount policy for large orders, please call us on 0532 706000.

- involve everyone;

- circulate the results;

- introduce aids to improve communication;

- design and conduct a programme of staff (and perhaps doctor) training;

- consult specialist books on human communication which provide useful material for staff training.

The practice manager should progress by repeating the questionnaire and interview exercise at appropriate intervals, perhaps every six months if improvement is required, and then maybe once a year, and circulate the results.

Aids to improve communication

These can include:

- a daybook for recording incoming messages (with a member of staff responsible for reviewing it during the day);

- colour coded memoranda forms (which may be no carbon required), to circulate a limited number of copies;

- labelled action trays for key staff with photocopying so that everyone gets a personal copy of important information;

- practice meetings with minutes taken for those who cannot attend;

- depending on the size of practice, up to four 'white-boards', visible only to practice staff, for births and deaths, hospital admissions and discharges, important notes and details of practice members who are away or on holiday. When wiping off entries, remember what people on holiday may need to know and make a note for them;

- informal 'blowing-off-steam' sessions from time to time, so that any communication problems can be aired and attended to without waiting for formal reviews.

Communications technology

Practice managers should ensure that appropriate technology is used

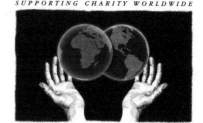
and that it is cost-effective. They should keep an eye on emerging technologies, as communications are developing with great speed.

Competition

The end of the communications monopoly previously enjoyed by the Post Office means that there is competition for the business of the practice. It is worth giving time to see the representatives of British Telecom, Mercury, the local TV cable company, power companies and any other communications companies offering services. Most will readily come in to review your communications needs and offer costed solutions. Encourage competition and get several quotations. The aim should be to identify opportunities to reduce existing costs as well as improving the service the practice receives.

NHS allowances

A careful study of the Red Book and relevant circulars, and a discussion with the family health service authority (FHSA) or Health Board, should alert you to any assistance which is available for funding communications developments.

Computers as communications tools

One of the least used functions of computers in medical practices is their communications function. Communications within a single practice building are made easier by networked computers which, depending on the software system in use, can provide facilities such as diary scheduling and mailbox. However, these are valuable only if everyone in the practice really wants to use them and is conscientious in doing so.

Communications with branch surgeries are possible through dial-up telephone modems which link computers, provided that there are measures to prevent unauthorised access. Leased lines can be used but are more expensive. For very busy links, consider asking British Telecom about ISDN (the integrated services digital network): it can be more economical than conventional telephone lines. Installation and line rental charges cost about £400 but the ISDN link has a much faster data throughput rate, data calls are much shorter and, depending on volume, call charges can be less.

Mobile communications

Pagers

The minimum mobile communications required by most doctors is a pager. This enables calls to be made to a central number for the pager device to receive a tone call or text message. Pagers can be leased or bought outright. For example, Hutchison Paging[1] offers pagers with a three-year warranty and a guaranteed replacement within two hours in the event of loss or malfunction. The simpler pagers are single or multi-tone, but those which can take a short message cost little more and should be considered. Pagers with an acknowledge facility, assuring the sender that the message has been received, are being developed.

It is worth getting quotations from several paging system companies to compare their costs and services. Theft of such devices poses no problems. The paging company will simply decline to accept calls if the device is reported stolen or the subscription payment lapses.

Mobile phones

These are essentially two-way radios that provide facilities similar to telephones. They can be bought direct from a manufacturer but there can be advantages in going to a company that offers a range, and deciding how much you want to pay. Cost depends on the facilities:

some mobile phones have more facilities than the doctors are ever likely to learn, remember or need. The costs of car mounting, if required, should be taken into account. There is a lot of competition in this market, and shopping around is advisable.

Messagers

Available only from Cognito Limited[2], these provide a two-way messaging service. They enable the doctor and the surgery staff, and anyone else equipped with the device, to key in messages and send them over a national wireless data network. A return signal indicates when a message is viewed. The 'control station' in the surgery or other health care facility can be a standard PC. The monthly airtime charge of £50 for each device pays for an unlimited number of messages. It is possible to send fax messages from them, and there is an incoming message voice bureau facility which enables people who do not have a messager to contact you. Depending on the volume of traffic, these devices can be less expensive to operate than mobile phones even though they cost some £600. Unlike mobile phones, it is not necessary to respond when a message arrives, thus reducing interruptions in consultations and meetings. This technology is increasingly used in organisations with mobile field forces, and it is only a matter of time before it catches on in the health and social services. It is an ideal communications medium for primary health care teams. Again, the company will 'disconnect' the messager if it is reported lost or stolen, or if the subscription payment lapses.

Radio modems

Instead of linking computers by telephone modems and land lines, it is possible to use radio modems and public wireless data networks (so-called because they are licensed by the DTI for public access). The main public wireless data networks are operated by RAM Mobile Data Ltd[3] and Cognito Limited. The radio modem is plugged into the RS232 port of the PC. Radio modems will soon be no larger than a thick credit card[4] which will fit into the slot in a small portable computer. They enable doctors, nurses and others to call patients' records by wireless into a portable notebook computer or notepad computer, and to make new entries and send them back to the surgery, thereby keeping the records constantly updated (the jargon is 'maintaining the record in real time'). The doctor will be able to know when the patient was last seen, by whom, what the clinical findings, treatment and prescribing were, and so on – very useful for duty doctors at weekends, for instance. This new technology minimises any risks which may arise when doctors visit patients without first seeing their medical records. It also makes it possible for prescriptions to be sent direct to the chemist by wireless link, so that patients do not have to wait for them to be dispensed.

Confidentiality

Doctors, practice managers and everyone in a practice must always ensure that medical confidentiality is preserved.

Conversations should not be overheard. If soundproofing is not good enough, improve it before something goes wrong, perhaps through an acoustic consultant.

Arrange computer screens to face away from windows or install venetian blinds; screens can not only be seen but can be picked up electronically from another building or a car.

Control access to computer systems, particularly at nights and weekends. If an intruder does get in, you can prevent access with password controls.

Remember that medical information sent by fax can go to an incorrectly dialled number or be seen by an unauthorised person at the destination.

Telephone calls and mobile telephone calls can be intercepted: GPs can, of course, use the telephone to discuss a case with a patient or a hospital, but discretion is required particularly if the information may provoke media interest or have commercial value.

Paper may not seem to be part of a communications system, but if old letters or records are found on a rubbish tip, you may soon realise that it is. Shredders do not cost much and guarantee that a practice will not get an unwelcome 'Medical records shock horror story' in the press.

References

1   Hutchison Paging (UK) Ltd, Senhouse Road, Darlington, Co Durham, DL1 4YG.
2   Cognito Limited, Newbury Business Park, London Road, Newbury, Berks RG13 2PZ.
3   RAM Mobile Data Ltd, Heathrow Boulevard, 280 Bath Road, West Drayton, Middx UB7 0DQ.

4 PCMCIA: Personal Computer Memory Card International Association, which sets standards for memory cards and devices which fit into slots in PCs.

Drawing up a Business Plan

Kathie Applebee

The definition of a business plan

The concept of producing a business plan is new to most general practitioners. Many feel alienated by the title and daunted by the task. Because of the word 'business', they think the plan has no place in general practice. As a result, many practices do indeed reject it.

It is important, therefore, to define the practice business plan, and to show the ways it resembles, and differs from, the annual report.

The annual report describes the practice and its patients, and any changes in activities and workload resulting from planned or imposed changes. It is a historical report of the preceding year.

The practice plan takes this a step further by attempting to forecast the growth of the practice, the changing requirements of its patients and the external forces which may affect both. It should include plans for dealing with these changes while reconciling the varying needs of the members of the primary health care team.

The financial element of the plan, which many regard as the hardest part, links the proposed plans for dealing with change with practice income and expenditure. Financial planning at practice level means setting budgets for spending and targets for income, and then working out how to achieve these.

Why produce a business plan?

Many family health service authorities (FHSAs) (and their equivalents in Scotland and Northern Ireland, the health boards) are requesting business plans from GPs. Plans produced at the request of external organisations should be done to their requirements, but if they do not

give any guidelines, the practice should focus on their needs and interests. For example, a business plan for a bank, if the practice is seeking a loan or overdraft, will differ from one for a regional authority or health board.

The latter plan would not be required to give financial information about the practice but would focus on morbidity figures, purchasing intentions, practice resources and premises, and details of the practice's clinical specialties. A bank, by contrast, would need to know the potential income of the practice, and would want detailed information about income and expenditure, financial management controls, and the assets of the practice.

Contents

The level of detail depends on those who produce the business plan. It should be sufficiently comprehensive to ensure that nothing important or relevant is overlooked, without going into unnecessary detail.

The contents should be a mixture of fact, forecast and opinion. The facts will include practical matters such as the size of the practice, the doctors' qualifications, experience and special interests, the numbers and types of staff, the size of premises and the like.

The forecasts or estimates will seek to anticipate changes to any of these, and to foresee external changes and constraints which may affect the practice.

Opinions about the practice can be invited from all members of the primary health care team, not just the partners and practice manager. Practice team members should be encouraged to describe what they like about the practice and what changes they would like to see. Involving practice members increases their sense of esteem and team membership, while the plan itself benefits from a wider and perhaps more balanced input. Involvement from the beginning will not only mean less work for whoever is producing the plan, but will also motivate those involved to ensure that the resulting plans are accurate and successful.

Timing

The practice may choose to update its business plan to coincide with the end either of its own financial year or with the NHS year. But these are both busy times and the plan can be updated as necessary, with a complete review at regular intervals to suit the practice. The important point is to treat the plan as a constantly changing guideline, not a fixed document which is filed away until the next annual review.

Distribution

Much depends on whether the plan was asked for by an outside agency and if practice team members were invited to contribute to it.

Plans for external organisations can be edited versions of the practice's own plan rather than completely different. For copyright reasons, copies distributed outside the practice should have the practice name and address on each page. The names of those on the distribution list should be listed on the front cover, which should signify clearly that it is a confidential document.

Copies can be given, at the practice's discretion, to anyone who has either contributed to the plan (the attached staff), who needs to know about the practice's current and future plans (the practice accountant), or has a right to know these things (the FHSA or health board general manager).

The layout

The following may be used as a guide and adapted to meet each practice's needs:

1 The mission statement

It is a popular practice to start plans with a paragraph which describes the practice philosophy. This is summed up by the day-to-day impression that the practice presents to patients, practice members and the local community.

Although this may appear at the beginning of the plan, it is best to devise it last of all, once the plan itself has given a clear picture of the practice and its potential.

2 The practice

This section encompasses the community and the practice's patients. It should include a brief history of the practice and describe the current state of events and future expectations.

- The history and evolution of the practice can affect its ability to attract new patients. A relatively new practice may lack traditional support, but a long-established practice may be so associated with certain areas that it finds it difficult to widen its practice boundaries to attract new patients.

- Community status and socio-economic, cultural and geographic factors will all affect the demands made on the practice. They must be monitored. The loss of a major employer in a small town will lead to economic hardship and associated ill-health. Cultural factors, such as more immigrant families, may result in a perceived need for more female doctors, nurses with family planning experience, voluntary or part-time interpreters, and so on. Physical factors, such as hard winters or patients living in remote areas, will affect the practice from time to time.

- Prevalent morbidity factors affect both the practice and the community. Plans will be needed to counter those which can be controlled or limited and should include expected changes, both good and bad, and the role of the practice in monitoring and influencing them.

3 Practice resources, which include people, equipment and money

These enable the practice to reach its primary goal of providing general medical services to its clients.

- General practitioners should state their personal details, professional qualifications and experience, and give relevant practice or personal goals (such as becoming a GP trainer).

- Staff should be listed by job title (and, optionally, by name), with brief details of each, including qualifications and experience. These details should include useful skills such as first aid qualifications, keyboard skills or languages.

- The practice premises should be described, highlighting good points and pointing out any defects which may act as constraints or prevent the practice from developing required services.

- Equipment details should include a list of specialised equipment, both clinical (e.g. an ECG machine) and administrative (e.g. computers, fax, mobile phones).

- Show the range of services on offer to patients and describe planned or potential changes.

4 External resources

- Details of secondary health care facilities should describe local and semi-local provider units (including those in the private sector), the quality of standards the practice requires them to have, and the referral patterns. Note any planned changes in referral patterns or usage of provider units.

- It should be shown whether social services play a supporting role or if they are overstretched and have, in effect, to be strengthened by practice resources.

- Describe other local services available to the practice and its patients.

- Fundholding practices should clearly describe changes to referral patterns and provider units which result from fundholding so that the regional health authority or health board can estimate the effect on local provider units.

5 Financial evaluation

- Income and expenditure: the contents and level of detail depend on what the plan is for. If it is chiefly for the benefit of the practice, it should be as detailed as possible. Obviously, a plan for a health body would not include details of practice finances unless information about certain areas (for example, improvements to the premises) is specifically requested.

  Useful detail will be added if someone in the practice can produce a budget for practice expenditure, targets for practice income, and cash flow forecasts to show when these will be paid out and received. Potential sources of additional income should also be described.

- The financial plans of fundholding practices should include their fundholding budget requirements, an assessment of provider pricing policies, the proposed expenditure of the management allowance, planned areas for savings and proposals for their use.

6 'SWOT' analysis

A 'SWOT' analysis is an assessment of the practice's Strengths, Weaknesses, Opportunities and Threats. These points come from the information collected in the preceding sections. Quite simply, rank every major item as either positive or negative, good or bad.

- **Strengths:** these include positive items that benefit patient care, produce extra income or attract patients.

- **Weaknesses:** it is helpful if the practice can be honest about its weaknesses because the business plan offers an opportunity to tackle these systematically and constructively. It may be helpful to list them in order of importance.

- **Opportunities:** are potential strengths which the practice should strive to acquire. They include under-used resources or forth-coming changes which could provide a chance to attract more patients or expand existing services.

- **Threats:** these include internal or external changes, such as staff leaving or new legislation, which may affect the practice adversely. Local practices may also be regarded as threats if they offer a service which is more attractive to your patients.

7 Goals and objectives

Once the strengths, weaknesses, opportunities and threats have been assessed, make relevant short-, medium- and long-term plans.

Every strength and opportunity needs a plan to enhance and improve it, while weaknesses and threats need plans to prevent or minimise harm to the practice.

All goals must be achievable and open to some form of audit or review to ensure that they are completed on time and according to budget to achieve the desired results. This approach will reduce the risk of woolly plans which lack goals, time scales or budgets.

Conclusion

End your practice plan on a strong positive note. Your mission statement is a statement of philosophy: it should conclude with a summary of the practical plans which are to be implemented or enhanced. These are designed to provide the infrastructure and services which will enable the practice to deliver the goals inherent in its mission statement.

The Legal Aspects of Health Practice Management

Angela Cullen

Medical records and their disclosure

General practice notes are technically owned by the relevant family health services authority and/or the Department of Health. The general practitioner is the custodian of the records and the only person with the right to decide whether they should be disclosed or not.

A general practitioner's medical records include hospital letters, medical reports, investigation results and so on. It is not necessary for a general practitioner to seek the consent of the various authors before releasing those records to the patient or to any third party.

The practice may get several requests for disclosure of a patient's medical records. Application for access may be made by:

1　the patient;
2　a person whom the patient has authorised in writing to apply;
3　a person who is responsible for a child (under 16), provided the child consents or cannot understand the meaning of the application;
4　a child, if old enough to understand the nature of the application;
5　a person appointed by a court to manage a patient's affairs, if the patient is mentally incapable;
6　the executor or next of kin of a deceased patient (though access should not be given if the patient while alive had given specific instructions against it);
7　any person who may have a claim arising out of the patient's death.

The Access to Health Records Act 1990 allows patients the right to see and/or have copies of any manual records made after 1 November 1991 and be given an explanation of them. It may however be necessary to disclose records made before then to enable the patient to understand what follows. Applications for access should be in writing and access given within 21 days, unless the records were written more than 40 days previously, which then allows 40 days for access.

The doctor may withhold access if serious harm to the patient's physical or mental health might result, or if the confidentiality of a third party may be breached. If the doctor agrees to a patient's request for inaccurate or incomplete information to be amended, he should do so but, if not, he must make a note of the conflict of views and give a copy to the patient. Penalties cannot be imposed by the courts in cases of disagreement but the courts can order the requirements of the Act to be fulfilled.

Computerised records

The Data Protection Act 1984 and the subsequent Order of 1987 on 'Modified Access to Personal Health Information' govern the patient's rights of access to personal data held on computer.

Patients have the right to be told by the doctor in general practice whether there is information about them held on computer, and to be supplied with copies of the information. There is no time limitation as in the Access to Health Records Act 1990. The application should be in writing and accompanied by the appropriate fee.

The time limit for disclosure is 40 days and normal routine updating is allowed to continue during this period. The doctor is allowed to withhold information as previously, where harm could be caused or a third person, other than a healthcare professional, could be identified.

The Courts may order payment of compensation for damage and any associated distress suffered by the patient as the result of lost, incorrect, inaccurate or misleading data.

Disclosure of children's records

Children over 16 years, and those under 16 years who are capable of understanding the significance of record disclosure, may give their own consent. If the child is not capable of giving consent, under the Provisions of the Children Act 1989 whoever has parental responsibility may consent. If married, the child's natural parents both have parental responsibility, but if unmarried only the mother has parental responsibility unless the father acquires it under other provisions of the Act.

Unless there is a Court Order to the contrary, either parent with parental responsibility may act independently and without consultation with the other parent. Court Orders may give parental responsibility to other people, such as grandparents or the local authority in certain situations.

Medical reports

The Access to Medical Reports Act 1988 and the Access to Personal Files and Medical Reports (Northern Ireland) Order 1991 give patients right of access to reports provided by the doctor (usually GP) who is or has been responsible for their medical treatment.

The Act defines care as 'examination, investigation or diagnosis for the purposes of, or in connection with, any form of medical treatment'. Reports prepared by independent medical examiners and occupational physicians who do not provide any clinical care are thus excluded from the Act's provisions.

The patient must be informed of his or her rights under the Act when requesting the report and must give consent. The patient will be asked if he or she wishes to see the report and the applicant (usually an insurance company or prospective employer) must notify the doctor of these wishes.

The onus is on the patient to make arrangements with the practice within 21 days, if he or she wishes to see the report, and it should not be submitted to the applicant until after that date. A copy must be retained by the practice for six months, during which time the patient must be allowed access if requested.

Access to the report can be withheld by the doctor, as previously stated, under the Access to Health Records Act 1990 and the Data Protection Act 1984 and the patient must be informed of this. The report must not be submitted if the patient withdraws his consent. If the patient disagrees with the content of the report, the doctor can amend it if he or she is in agreement, but if not, must attach the patient's own comments to the report. The Courts cannot impose penalties in cases of disagreement but can order the requirements of the Acts to be fulfilled.

Insurance companies often ask for information about deceased patients. Information may only be given with the informed consent of the executor to the estate or next of kin if the patient died intestate. In deciding whether information should be released, the doctor should take into account the likely wishes of the deceased.

Disclosure to solicitors

Solicitors' requests for disclosure of patients' records are becoming more common in general practice. If the solicitor states clearly that he or she is acting for the patient, the written consent of the patient is not strictly necessary.

If the doctor delays disclosure and is uncooperative, the solicitor may apply for a Court Order under Section 34 of the Supreme Court Act 1981, which provides for the compulsory release of records once a writ against the primary defendant has been issued. If successful, the doctor who has resisted disclosure unreasonably may find the costs of the application awarded against him or her.

If the request for disclosure is made by a third party, the defendant's solicitor, for instance, the records should not be disclosed without the patient's written permission. If disclosure is withheld due to lack of consent from the patient, the doctor would not be likely to have the costs of an application for a Court Order awarded against him or her, as he or she would be safeguarding patient's interests and confidentiality.[1]

Confidentiality

The GP and his or her staff have a duty of confidentiality to patients which extends beyond the grave. It is important for patients to have this trust in the practice in order to speak freely and impart information.

If confidentiality is breached, the patient has several ways of seeking redress:

1 He or she may apply to the courts for an injunction or a civil claim for damages. For civil damages to be awarded the patient must prove:

   (a) a duty of confidentiality;
   (b) a breach of that duty;
   (c) damage has resulted as a consequence.

2 An alleged breach of confidentiality can be referred to a Professional Conduct Committee of the General Medical Council for doctors or the UKCC for nurses, or

3 To the family health services authority, though a breach of confidentiality may not contravene the GP's Terms of Service.

Legal requirements for release of information

1 Under the Public Health (Infectious Disease) Regulations 1968, certain infectious diseases must be notified. This is a statutory requirement and failure to comply is a criminal offence.

2 A doctor who has reasonable grounds to suspect a patient is addicted to a drug scheduled in the Misuse of Drugs (Notification and Supply to Addicts) Regulations 1985 must inform the Chief Medical Officer of the Home Office Drugs Branch.

3 A doctor treating a patient with a terminal illness must provide the Registrar of Deaths with the Certificate of Death stating, inter alia, the cause of death.

4 A doctor or midwife present at birth must inform the District Health Authority of that birth (or stillbirth) within 36 hours (NHS Notification of Births and Deaths Regulations 1974).

5 Under the Abortion Act 1967, a practitioner terminating a pregnancy must notify the Chief Medical Officer of the Department of Health or the Scottish Home & Health Department.

Police

The Police have no statutory right to inspect records without the patient's consent, whatever offence has been committed.

Under the Road Traffic Act 1972, the GP is obliged to supply the name and address only, no clinical information, which may lead to the identification of the driver of a vehicle who is alleged to be guilty of an offence under the Act.

The Prevention of Terrorism (Temporary Provisions) Act 1989 obliges the GP to supply information which may help to prevent, or lead to the apprehension of a person involved in, an act of terrorism.

The Police and Criminal Evidence Act 1984 provides wide-ranging powers of entry, search and seizure. Circuit judges may order that the police be given medical records to inspect or take away. The most important condition is that the documents are likely to be of substantial value to the investigation of a serious arrestable offence.

Coroner

The Coroner (Procurator Fiscal in Scotland) has powers to investigate sudden, suspicious or unexplained deaths. Information should be disclosed to a coroner to allow him or her to determine whether an inquest should be held.

Courts

A doctor must obey a subpoena compelling him or her to attend court or to produce confidential documents. A doctor cannot claim special privilege as a witness before a court or tribunal. He or she may appeal to the judge or chairman, but if directed to answer a question, may be found in contempt of court if he or she fails to do so.

Disclosure of information on the grounds of public interest

The General Medical Council's guidelines (paragraph 86) on confidentiality specifically mention that doctors, when deciding whether to disclose information, should take into account whether 'the failure to disclose appropriate information would expose the patient, or someone else, to a risk of death or serious harm'.

Aids/HIV positive patients

Aids is not a statutorily notifiable disease. Disclosure of clinical details without the patient's consent to a third party is permitted only when the doctor judges that failure to disclose would put the health of any of the healthcare team at serious risk, or to safeguard such persons (spouse or sexual partner) from a possibly fatal infection (GMC, May 1988).

Research and clinical trials

With increasing emphasis on medical audit, it is important to remember the duty of confidentiality. If information about patients is to be disclosed for the purpose of medical teaching, research or audit, and the patient can be identified, that patient's consent must be obtained.

Children at risk

Where a healthcare worker has reasonable grounds to suspect child abuse, his or her paramount responsibility and duty are with the infant patient and it is perfectly legitimate to supply information (whether orally or in writing) to the appropriate authorities to ensure that the child is protected.[2]

Minor surgery and consent to treatment

GPs are encouraged under the new contract to provide minor surgery for their patients. Oral consent is adequate for most minor surgical procedures in general practice but it must be obtained by the doctor and not delegated to another healthcare professional. The fact that consent has been obtained should be recorded in the patient's records, together with any warnings or details of possible complications given. The post-operative arrangements should also be explained and any allergies recorded.

It would be more appropriate to obtain written consent in some cases, such as from parents of children under 16, and for vasectomy.

Histology

It is recommended that every excised lesion should be sent to the laboratory for histological examination. It is the responsibility of the practice to ensure that a report is received for every specimen sent for examination and the appropriate action taken.[3]

Product liability

The Consumer Protection Act 1987 requires a producer to ensure that a product is up to standard and fit for the intended purpose.[4]

Liability for damage caused to a patient rests with the producer or supplier. General practitioners become suppliers when they dispense any product to a patient, particularly suture material or local anaesthetics when performing minor surgery. It is therefore important for GPs to maintain records which identify the producer of a product or the name of the supplier, to avoid liability.

To do this, a record of the name of the product, the batch number, the supplier and the date the product was used, should be kept for ten years and four months.

A patient may suffer damage from a defect in a piece of equipment, such as a nebuliser on loan or a surgical instrument, during the course of treatment. The liability rests with the producer or supplier of the equipment but they may escape liability if it can be shown that the equipment was not maintained or calibrated or used in accordance with the instructions. It is therefore essential that equipment, the autoclave, for instance, is properly maintained.

Vaccines and drugs must be stored correctly and at temperatures stipulated by the manufacturers, and accurate records kept.

The Health & Safety at Work Act 1974 requires that maintenance of equipment is carried out.

References

1 Can I see the records? P J Hoyte MDU
2 Confidentiality. C O'Donovan MDU
3 Minor Surgery. P B Dando MDU
4 Medico-Legal Aspects of Practice Nursing S Parker & C Wilson MDU

Part Two

Human Resource Management

Managing People

Merrill Whalen

Setting the scene

There can be little doubt that general medical practice is both busy and complex. The pace of change is greater than ever before. For some, it is an exciting time, meeting every new challenge with enthusiasm and determination to succeed; for others, the realisation that roles and responsibilities have to be analysed, amended, sometimes changed completely, brings feelings of insecurity, uncertainty and threat.

Nonetheless, most health care professionals and consumers (our patients) will extol the virtues of an improved primary care service where the emphasis is on 'planning' (although the means by which all is achieved is often in question and debate).

The major hurdle for general practice is that the 'new, improved, planned service' is integral with the traditional 'reactive service'. It would therefore seem that the quart-into-a-pint-pot scenario is with us for some time.

Identifying health needs and the painstaking but necessary task of balancing these needs with available resources is serious business indeed.

General medical practitioners are caring family physicians with responsibilities for the medical, social and psychological welfare of their patients as individuals, of families and of the community at large. Yet, modern practice demands far more than that. Whether new responsibilities are welcomed or shunned, wholly believed in or viewed with suspicion, the reality is that real progress, moving the practice forward in a way that is both efficient and effective (there is a difference), can begin when:

- aims and objectives are fully discussed, agreed, written down in

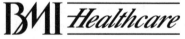

BMI HEALTHCARE AND PARTNERSHIPS IN CARE LTD: A HEALTHY MARKET SHARE

The resources offered by BMI Healthcare, the independent acute care provider, and its sister organisation for psychiatric services, Partnerships in Care Ltd, ensure a healthy market share.

With 1,417 beds, BMI provides 13 per cent of private acute care beds in the UK. Partnerships in Care provides 392 beds for mentally ill, handicapped and brain injured patients.

BMI's chain of 18 hospitals stretches from Canterbury to Glasgow. It includes The Harley Street Clinic, The Princess Grace Hospital and The Portland Hospital in the capital, and the largest private hospital outside London, Manchester's 180-bed Alexandra.

BMI acquired two 'NHS partnership' hospitals recently: Bishops Wood, partnering Mount Vernon, Northwood, Middlesex, and The Runnymede Hospital, sharing a site with St Peter's, Chertsey, Surrey. These are in addition to BMI's original 'partnership' hospital in Chesterfield.

Some 100,000 patients are admitted to BMI hospitals annually, and 250,000 are seen as outpatients. Surgery ranges from day case procedures to heart surgery, neurosurgery and organ transplantation. The most modern technology is provided, and the services are backed by resident doctors, intensive care units and the most sophisticated medical facilities available.

Under-use of special equipment and staff imposes cost penalties. To help both public and private hospitals avoid downtime costs, European Healthcare Associates Group, a BMI Healthcare subsidiary, provides mobile magnetic resonance imaging, cardiac catheterisation and lithotripsy services.

Trading as Healthlinx, in a joint initiative with Private Patients Plan (PPP), BMI Health Services offers healthcare services to industry and health screening to companies and individuals. Healthlinx has headquarters in London and a chain of 13 screening centres, from Winchester to Glasgow.

BMI Healthcare's facilities include Medical Diagnostic Laboratories, a central London-based unit, handling major acute clinical pathology. MDL offers hospitals and general practitioners year-round, 24-hour laboratory services with full clinical support. As well as providing a comprehensive autologous blood service, MDL performs some 20,000 crossmatches each year and a million chemistry, haematology and microbiology tests. Major clients include pharmaceuticals companies and government services.

Partnerships in Care Ltd's first unit, Kneesworth House, was opened in 1985 at Bassingbourn cum Kneesworth, Cambridgeshire. It is a hospital, with 151 beds, and the administrative headquarters of Partnerships in Care. Work focuses on the assessment, treatment and rehabilitation of disturbed and mentally disordered adults, mostly referred from NHS authorities lacking appropriate facilities. Stockton Hall, in Yorkshire, offers similar services.

Diversification into head and brain injury treatment led to the opening of Grafton Manor, in Northamptonshire. Its success resulted in the formation of Brain Injury Services, which enables patients to prepare for independent living, while receiving professional support.

The Old Rectory, near Diss, Norfolk, accommodates adults with severe learning disabilities. Nearby, at Palgrave, St John's House provides clinical assessment and treatment of adults with moderate learning disabilities, whose behaviour is too challenging for NHS facilities.

In Wales, Llanarth Court, near Abergavenny, provides 62 beds for mentally ill patients and adults with mild learning disabilities.

a practical, easily understood way, monitored regularly and evaluated. (If you don't define a route, then any old route is bound to be OK.)

- sound business principles are applied. Many doctors remain uneasy about the relationship between financial aspects of their practice and the delivery of health care. ('I'm proud to wear my doctor hat, but isn't it a bit unethical to wear a business/financial one?') Just as well-organised medical records can take a portion of credit for good care of patients, so can the financially buoyant practice that maximises income, monitors and controls expenditure – and what's unethical about that?

- working towards a communication culture – that goes far beyond the weekly meeting scenario.

- above all, managing people successfully . . . the greatest resource of all, human energy!

This chapter considers people. It provides a short practical guide to key issues, based on the author's experience as practice manager in a large, progressive general medical practice in a particularly deprived area of Edinburgh, and in full-time training (organisation and management for medical receptionists, practice managers and general practitioners).

People come first

People must come first. They should be an organisation's most prized asset.[1]

Profit through people, not at the expense of them. Consider people as a prized asset, not a variable. In this context, the reader must see 'profit' not only in traditional financial terms, but as improved service, effectiveness and benefits to primary health care team, patients and colleagues. GP principals individually and as the partnership clearly 'carry the can' for implementation of the new contract or for leading the practice towards fundholding, but in most cases, staff members carry the administrative burden that will lead to that achievement.

Administration and Organisation –DOES
Management – ACHIEVES

Many people have made a lot of money going on about general management, managing people, writing books, expounding theories and jargon until it is coming out of your ears, and running courses and more courses. Sometimes, it is even suggested that it would be impossible to be an effective manager without passing psychometric tests, assessments and high level degrees. Training matters, but so does experiential learning. Research-based practice matters, but so does common sense – it's just that sometimes it's not that common!

Good managers, be they an appointed practice manager or a GP who manages the practice, must be:

- Enthusiastic

- Committed

- Above average in communication skills, and

- Intelligent, of course!

The nuts and bolts of general practice management or official systems of the health service can then be learned.

Management is often used interchangeably with leadership. Some writers have tried to draw the distinction, but most practising managers accept that they are much the same. Leadership is an elusive concept, a word often used loosely with little apparent understanding of what it means. According to Sir Michael Edwardes, 'Success is about leadership and leadership is about success'[2]. That tells us little about leadership, yet has a ring of truth.

What do we really mean, therefore, when we say that 'he/she is a good manager/leader of people'? If you ask a friend or colleague what he thinks leadership is, the usual response is to ponder, identify a national or world-renowned leader and list qualities rather than actually explain what leadership is.

If good leadership of people is only to do with qualities, honesty, integrity, dependability, trust, initiative, self-assurance, compassion and so on, there would be little hope for most managers. But if we think of leadership as the management of people, it's less elusive, easier to grasp.

Many organisations throughout the United Kingdom have registered commitment and are currently working towards a national standard of good practice.[3] But when the socio-economic climate is still one of recession, business is struggling to survive. So why bother with a national standard?

One hallmark of well-run companies is the way they treat their customers. They produce products that work first time, provide service, are responsive to customers and have consistently high standards.

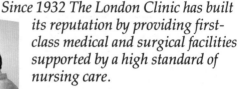

Dig deeper and you find that the same companies are the ones which also treat their employees well and get the best out of them. They train and develop employees, they have good management–staff relations, employees perform well and the business runs smoothly and successfully.

The best companies recognise that their success depends critically on employees and their skills. Staying competitive, remaining profitable and surviving in an increasingly competitive world all depend on getting the best out of people and continually improving their skills.

- teamwork at all levels of the organisation;

- getting things right first time, with fewer errors, less waste and fewer costs;

- optimising the use of computers and technology;

- treating customers well and being responsive to their needs.

Employees therefore expect companies to develop their skills. People are no longer prepared to accept poor management or inadequate training and development. If things are not right, the best people will move to companies which do these things better.

'But that's all to do with industry and commerce – we're different!' Substitute 'health care' for 'product', 'practice' for 'business or organisation', 'patients and colleagues' for 'customers', 'best practice and standard setting' for 'competitive', and it is clear that there is no difference.

At this point, you may well think this is confirming what you know already:

'Good leadership is about managing people'
'People are your organisation'
'People matter'
'You have to invest in your people'

Let me relate what usually happens at the end of a training course. Delegates are asked to think quietly and then commit to paper several action points. 'What are *you* going to do, or do differently when you go into your respective practice, tomorrow?' asks the trainer.

'Well,' comes the reply, 'I am going to communicate better with my staff,' and next: 'for me, this course has heightened my awareness that staff need to be more involved'. Or, 'the main thing for me is to delegate more.'

At this point the trainer takes control: 'Sorry, this tells me nothing.

A lot of easily said words, that is all.' What action, what *specific* thing, are you going to do?

The following can only be read in terms of 'helpful hints' and is not definitive. Theory and any academic approach are now left behind.

Let us see what you can, practically, do to lead and manage the people for whom you have responsibility. What is fundamental? What is important? What seems to work?

Laying sound foundations

As a manager, you will have responsibilities for appointing new staff. There are three main aspects to this:

1 deciding what jobs you need new staff for;
2 deciding what sort of people you will need to fill these jobs;
3 how to find such people.

Selection and recruitment procedures and the skills needed to ensure you get the best person for the job would require volumes to detail. The following points should provide a framework.

- A full analysis of the job.

  This should be conducted long before you think about the job advertisement. Is there a vacancy? Is this an opportunity for change? Is there a more creative or alternative way to get the work undertaken and goals achieved? Should job descriptions move from simply being lists of tasks to include purpose, responsibility, expected results, standards expected?

- Describing the person for the job.

  Being clear about the 'must have' skills and qualities and the 'would be nice to have'. Simple and basic, but look around and see where blatant mistakes have been made.

- Getting suitable applicants.

  Too vague or brief an advertisement may only add to your workload of sorting out unsuitable applications.

- Dealing with applications

  Is there a system to deal with this?

- Interviewing

Preparation, structure the interview, protect time, evaluate the interview. If you feel you do not have time for all this, it will be nothing compared to the time spent if you get it wrong.

An attractive though all too often disastrous alternative is to invite 'Mrs. Green – a little part-time job will be good for her' – have you heard that before? Beware! You are the professional, and stand your ground. You have a practice to run, a major responsibility that demands staff of high calibre.

- Induction

  This is another cornerstone to get firmly in place. Watch out for the pitfalls of 'Learning from Nellie', or, worse still, 'You'll soon get the hang of it'.

- Induction programme

  This provides a great opportunity, and is time well spent. The return on your investment can prove excellent. A checklist might include:

  - some historical background;
  - aims and objectives (and where exactly the new employee fits in);
  - system and services;
  - current difficulties and concerns;
  - terms and conditions of service, including employees' rights;
  - rules and regulations (including house rules or unofficial arrangements);
  - standards expected (eg 'In our practice, standards mean that you answer the telephone in a particular way') – spell it out;
  - training and development opportunities;
  - appraisal system.

  The effective manager will have to consider:

  - the structure and the length of time required for induction;
  - back-up printed information;

- who supervises the induction programme;
- how you assess how the new trainee is doing.

Keep it simple, be committed, and make it happen.

At the beginning of this chapter, we touched on some of the changes and the planning we need to be effective. Primary care, and indeed all disciplines involved in health care, are being encouraged to look carefully at what they are doing and their monitoring, recording and evaluating of information.

Clinical, medical and organisational audit, health needs assessment, business plans, operational plans and practice annual reports are a lot of work but make good sense if resources are to go where the need is.

Involve staff

Staff members must be involved and have to know about plans. Otherwise, they aimlessly busy themselves in a task-oriented environment. Would you be interested in counting numbers at the end of each surgery or clinic if no-one ever told you why?

That peaks and troughs of workload can be monitored and that clear factual information enables doctors and managers to take management decisions, is a revelation to most medical receptionists.

That quality information about systems, services and research is the lifeblood of primary care, and paves the way forward, suddenly adds a new perspective to an otherwise boring job. Would you be interested in fees and forms and meticulous systems if you were unaware of the independent contractor status of the general practitioner?

Experience in working closely with staff from the general medical practice still indicates the vast majority do not fully understand the GP's independent contractor status. Quite simply, staff have to know 'why' to enable them to work effectively, with enthusiasm and commitment, towards a common goal.

But involvement extends beyond knowing what is going on. Involvement has been described as the process of securing commitment. Staff members will be much more inclined to believe in decisions and support them when their views and ideas have been sought. It takes very little on the part of the managers to ask, 'Do you have any ideas on how we might improve the system?' but it will mean a great deal to the employees.

Regular feedback is essential if this line of enquiry is to be taken seriously, and to maintain credibility. The key here is regular, honest dialogue that accepts and respects opinions and ideas, where everyone is valued for the contribution they can bring. Can you think of some projects you have on the go at the moment? Set them out on paper and against each put the names of everyone, or groups of people, who will be affected, even in a small way. Is everyone (or a representative from each group) aware of the objective and the plan? If not, take action now.

If stakeholders are uninformed and uninvolved, that is, they 'find out' in due course that they have extra work to do, they may well prove uninterested and uncooperative.

Value staff

There is a common misconception that money is a prime motivator, that nothing else matters as long as you can pay high wages. But research shows that this is not so. Money does matter, of course, but again, it should be seen as a cornerstone and got right in relation to skills, experience and personal qualities.

That will get people into post and ensure that they come to work but it is unlikely to have any effect on true effectiveness and development. The skilled manager finds out what makes each employee 'tick', the psychological contract with their job of work. Is it sole ownership of a piece of work? Is it group activity? Is it responsibility? Is it contributing to the social good? Is it being developed to maximum capacity? Is it routine, methodical, detailed work?

In one piece of research which investigated what bosses thought their staff would say and what employees did actually say the following findings emerged:

Job Factors	Employee	Bosses
* 1 most important, 10 least important		
Full appreciation of work done	1	8
Feeling of being in on things	2	10
Sympathetic help with personal problems	3	9
Job security	4	2
Good wages	5	1
Interesting work	6	5
Promotional growth in organisation	7	3
Personal loyalty to employees	8	6
Good working conditions	9	4
Tactful discipline	10	7

Source: Le Due (1980)

This is completely borne out by primary care staff. 'We want to know what is going on and be involved'; 'We want to be valued and appreciated' are the two issues most often raised when working with receptionists, managers and GP principals themselves.

Sometimes, feeling valued derives from a simple and sincere 'thank-you'. Not the 'you're great', 'thanks a million', 'can't do without you' that some people trot out. These have little meaning. Picking up the phone to say 'thank-you' to someone who has put themselves out for you, writing a note, celebrating completion of success at the end of a project, such as meeting targets, are what I have in mind.

'Managing' patients

Managers should see their role as central to patient care, and not in a restricted way. The challenge is to manage an entire practice list while also nurturing and maintaining a culture, philosophy and service that ensures each individual patient feels special and valued. If management is about achievement, then every little helps. If you want to change things, 'ca canny', as they say north of the border, or 'walk before you run'. Aims and objectives must be realistic, achievable and measurable, but certainly do not have to be sophisticated – the simpler the better.

In conclusion, lecturers know that only 10 per cent at best of the information they impart will be retained by their listeners. If the same is so for this chapter, let it be:

People are the most important asset you have;
Get the 'right' people on board;
Invest in them;
Involve them;
Value them.

How you do that is up to you – is it not that very fact that makes management exciting and challenging?

References

1   *Superboss – The A–Z of Managing People Successfully* David Freemantle (Gower Publishing Group)
2   Sir Michael Edwardes (Goldsmith & Clutterbuck, 1984; 13)
3   Investors in People Scotland (Glasgow Development Agency)

Building a Practice Team

Susie Lawson

General practice should provide the best possible care for the community it serves. Since the introduction of the National Health Service, partnerships have developed from one or two doctors to five or six partners and in some cases more. There has also been a huge increase in the number of administrative staff. Where there were perhaps a couple of part-time receptionists (often the doctor's wife), there are now 15 or 20 administrative staff in bigger practices, including practice managers, secretaries and receptionists. Now surgeries are seldom held in the doctor's front room, but in modern health and medical centres, with nurses, health visitors and midwives holding their own clinics. More community services are developing a practice base in such fields as physiotherapy, chiropody, speech therapy, psychology, psychiatry, social services and counselling. With the rise of community-based services comes the need to develop a practice team in which everyone can employ his or her particular knowledge and skills and where an atmosphere can be created for everyone to understand and value each other's work.

Members of a practice need to act as an integrated unit, not as separate individuals with unrelated roles. Their concern should be for the success of the practice team rather than their own individual functions.[1]

Where to start

Developing a practice team may seem a simple matter but in fact is complicated, and success may not come easily. Team building involves bringing together many disciplines which in the past have worked in isolation and within their own hierarchical structures. Bringing the team together and seeking their opinions on how to identify barriers and merge positions is the first and most crucial part of the development of the practice team. It can be done either at a series of meetings within the practice or on an 'away day' somewhere outside the practice. Either method takes a lot of preparation and organisation.

Who will be included?

Obviously, those who work and have their base within the health centre should be included, but who else? It is up to the practice to decide, and the team may gradually develop from a core of people to include more and more specialties, but the decision can create conflict before the meeting has even begun. Communication between members and potential members of the team is important and plans should be explained in advance of team building meetings.

Where will it be held?

Clinical staff are often interrupted during meetings within the practice, which can be very disruptive to team building exercises. It is therefore advisable to hold this meeting in the evening, on the practice half day or at a weekend. An 'away day', preferably with an overnight stay, is a good way of getting everyone to relax and to see their colleagues as individuals rather than in terms of their role or their uniform.

The questions to ask

- Where are we now?
- Where do we want to be?
- How will we get there?
- How will we know when we get there?

Ask the staff about the practice goals and do a critical analysis of the *real* situation. The practice goal will probably be to provide the best service for its patients, but then ask how the practice team can achieve that goal and measure its progress.

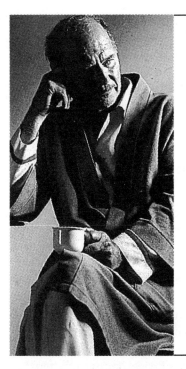
SHEFFIELD PATHOLOGY SERVICES

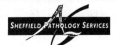

What appears from the outside to be a good team may have hidden problems. Those organising the meeting or 'away day' must watch for undercurrents and deal with delicate situations promptly and carefully, ever mindful of the concerns of those involved. There may be a need to go back to square one to get the team to understand the implications, opportunities and difficulties arising from recent changes in the NHS.

Meetings and away days

Many family health service authorities (FHSAs) are willing to help, and specific outside professional help can be obtained. Facilitators should be experienced and able to keep everyone on track. They should ensure that dominant members are kept under control and should draw opinions from the quieter members of the team. It is also important before and during the meeting to impress upon reception staff that they, too, are part of the team and that their views matter if the practice is to make changes in future. Ideally, an agenda should be agreed in advance. If the assembled team is large, it can be broken into smaller groups that should include representatives from each department. People who would feel overawed in large meetings, even with their own friends and colleagues, will often speak freely to smaller, informal groups. These can nominate a spokesperson who can feed back its thoughts to the rest of the practice.

Everyone should be able to say exactly what he or she thinks and know that no offence will be taken. That may, however, cause ill-feeling rather than solve problems if it is not handled diplomatically. The team may need to evolve for quite a time before members are relaxed enough to do this.

In the end, everyone must be clear about the decisions that have been taken and any doubts must be resolved.

Difficulties in team building

'Letting go' of particular tasks by doctors and clinical staff is a similar problem to delegation, but can be more difficult for individuals to accept. Litigation has made it more difficult for doctors to pass on medical care to others in the team and their sense of responsibility and confidentiality is often in conflict with team building ideals. Nurses, health visitors and practice nurses may also find problems in the role-sharing exercise. Any overlap of roles should be addressed by those involved: management can point out difficulties but the solutions lie with them. If they can discuss their roles, appreciate their respective professional skills, be open and flexible and supportive to each other, then the team building exercise is working. Joint training is one way of introducing the practice team concept and encouraging doctors and nurses to discuss clinical problems openly. The new postgraduate educational allowance regulations[3] can be used to promote joint learning opportunities within the practice and outside it.

Motivating everyone to become involved in change can be hard work and some members of the team may dislike holding meetings outside working hours. They should be encouraged to share their ideas and to be involved in the development of the practice. Suggestions should always be followed up even if only to explain why they are impracticable.

Suggestions at any meeting should be addressed there and then, because it is all too easy for doctors and staff to have a good idea and expect someone else, usually the practice manager, to set the wheels in motion. New ideas and working methods should include quality circles and audit[2] which, if properly executed, are very time-consuming. Practice managers must be honest about what they can do, to avoid becoming overloaded with extra work.

Further meetings often transpire from 'away days'. It may be agreed to develop smaller working groups with their own special responsibilities. That is a good idea, with groups comprising representatives from each relevant department. Meetings, however, entail more time, which is already at a premium. Minutes of meetings can be circulated, but these are usually scanned or even 'binned' by those not involved in the group. It may, therefore, be easier for each member to be responsible for telling his or her department about decisions and progress. The communications between teams are vital factors which affect team development.

⚠ Factors affecting team development

Change

The team building exercise involves cultural changes within the practice. Reasons for this cultural change should be explained and understood by all those involved.[3] The Griffiths Report[4] stated that resources coming into the NHS would not keep up with the demands of the community. With the changing role of community care and more patients being discharged from hospitals earlier, it is no longer a matter of maintaining present services; money and time must be available to develop and improve community care. There is also a steady rise in the number of elderly patients who need the services of several members of the practice team.

The need to adapt to change must be accepted by the practice manager and the effects of decisions monitored carefully to ensure that the benefits are realised. Change handled well can motivate and stimulate, and should create a comfortable situation. Handled badly, however, it will cause anger, mistrust, resentment and conflicts of opinion which are difficult to handle.

Communications

The manager should set up and monitor effective communication systems. Methods of communicating vary and depend on the structure of the practice. Regular or daily verbal contact can aid team development, but some doctors may remain reluctant to discuss or delegate care.

Memos need to be kept short. Most people will read one page, scan two pages and leave three or more pages to read later!

Meetings will only succeed with a definite agenda and organised chairmanship. Notice boards in common rooms have been found useful by some practices but one person should be responsible for tidying and removing notices. Message books may be appropriate but need to be kept in a prominent place and initialled when read.

Team building exercise

Tackle a common task which will involve as many of the disciplines as possible, including secretaries and receptionists in the discussions as, being the first line of contact, they need to know a lot of detail.

Examples of tasks which could be tackled as a team building exercise include:

1 The development of an asthma clinic

- doctor and nurse can receive their initial training together;
- secretaries and receptionists can be involved in setting up the appointments system;

- computer operators can develop input procedures and a call and recall system;

- health visitors and school nurses can provide information and support to schools and families.

2 Introduction of a smoking cessation clinic

- initial discussions about who would be targeted, or if it should be open for all interested patients, can involve doctors, nurses, health visitors, school nurses and midwives;

- the running of the clinic can bring together any of the disciplines and can also have some psychological or psychiatric nurse input if the group feels that they could benefit from some stress management training.

Conclusions

The changes which are taking place in the National Health Service in the 1990s offer a real chance for the development of a structured primary health care team.

In most situations, it is difficult to instigate change, but the present climate in the health service, with the emphasis changing to community care, presents an exciting prospect for those who are willing to accept the challenge and promote the introduction of a practice team. This, in turn, should improve patient care in the community.

References

1 RCGP Quality in General Practice – Policy Statement 2 November 1985
2 Irvine D and Irvine S (eds.), *Making Sense of Audit*. Radcliffe Medical Press Oxford 1991
3 Handy C, *Understanding Organizations* (chapter 7). Penguin Business Library 1985
4 NHS Management Inquiry 1983

Training

Trevor Illsley

Introduction

Doctors in general practice are constantly using medical jargon such as 'LMP', 'TFT', 'GFR' and 'highly selective vagotomy'. They have spent most of their formative years learning and thinking along such lines, and was part of their principal goals when they embarked on their careers. After all, years of training to gain this knowledge is essential to treat demanding patients and provide the best possible care for an ageing population.

However, during the late 1980s the Government stated its intention that the NHS would be judged on its ability to make the best use of available resources to provide quality of service and value for money. A series of White Papers followed, starting in 1987 with *Promoting Better Health*. This laid the foundation for the new GP contract. Later came *Working For Patients*, which contained recommendations for far-reaching changes in the structure and management of the NHS and the *National Health Service and Community Care Bill*, followed in 1990 by the new GP contract itself.

Going commercial

During this time, a new type of jargon began to emerge which made many community doctors ill at ease. Independent medical advisors and indicative prescribing amounts came in, together with business planning, mission statements, fundholding and so on. More commercial terms took their place alongside the familiar medical jargon and business pressures became apparent in general practice. Also, practice managers were being placed, some from within surgeries and others from outside the NHS.

Need for new training

The pharmaceutical company Glaxo is the largest supplier of medicines to the NHS in value terms, but also provides other services in the form of educational grants, donations to hospital departments and the funding of medical symposia. During this time of rapid change in the NHS, the company also saw the need for another service, training on the business and management side of general practice. To provide this, we had first to determine what form it should take. Should it, for example, be aimed primarily at GPs themselves or at practice managers? The first step was a detailed training needs analysis (TNA). At this stage, a training company, Infocus Skills Ltd, and a specialist medical education consultancy, Knowledge House Ltd, were recruited. The TNA involved detailed discussions with doctors, practice managers and family health service authorities to see where they felt the need for more training was as a result of the changes that were taking place. It became clear that it was not only medical practitioners who needed training, but the practice as a whole.

Training needs

Several common features came out of the TNA. These were

- business and management skills are becoming increasingly important;
- the whole practice needs attention;
- the potential costs of training are a barrier;
- courses offered vary in quality and relevance;
- the real problem is how to plan and initiate the right programme, apply the lessons learnt and sustain development.

The practice as a business

There appeared to be four main areas to address in order to help practices run their businesses. Initially, therefore, the four modules were as follows.

1 The practice as a business

Presenting business and finance concepts in a way that is relevant to those managing a practice. This is chiefly aimed at partners who do not have specific financial responsibility or expertise but would like to play a greater role within the practice.

2 Resource utilisation

Presenting concepts and practical activities to improve practice efficiency using the two key resources – people and time. There are two versions of this course, for partners and practice managers respectively.

3 Managing staff performance

Presenting core 'people management concepts' that are at the heart of successful organisations. This provides practical experience through syndicate work and role play and allows for specific action plans for practice staff.

4 Train the trainer for patients first

Provides training for practice managers in customer care skills and how to train others within the practice.

Each of these modules was developed to run as a day course and involves six to eight delegates. The relatively small numbers mean that all sessions can be interactive and the day tailored to individual needs.

A programme based solely or heavily on management skills for GPs only will have a slow uptake. This is because GPs took up a career in medicine to treat patients clinically and only some, probably those in large or fundholding practices, are interested in management as such. The rest are interested to some extent, primarily for financial reasons, but all could be encouraged to appreciate how good management can benefit them personally and the practice as a whole, by creating more time for them to practise medicine and gain more income.

Practice 2000

Once the four modules had been developed, the service was given its own identity – Practice 2000. Six experienced representatives were taken from Glaxo Laboratories' sales force and trained on the content and delivery of the modules. The response to a pilot scheme was excellent and the programme was rolled out.

Feedback

An important aspect of the training modules as they developed was feedback from attendees. That gives delegates an opportunity to evaluate the sessions, comment on personal objectives achieved and decide on the most useful parts of the course, any changes they recommend, the quality of the instruction and any further development needed. It is from these evaluation forms that we maintain our needs-based training programme. From this emerged a demand for shorter sessions within surgeries to include other members of staff such as receptionists, secretaries and nursing staff.

Role of practice managers

As in any successful business, relevant training is needed not only by the managers but also by those being managed. To provide these in-surgery sessions meant that we had to discuss individual training needs with practice managers. To get a whole practice together with minimal disruption from patients and telephones is not easy, so sometimes an hour after evening surgery has been allocated to staff training. Subjects covered in these sessions have included communication skills or 'handling difficult patients', for example.

Practice 2000 is now being organised regionally across the UK and continues to be successful. Strategy 2000 is also being developed. This includes computer software based around the rules and regulations of the Red Book.

Part Three

Financial Planning

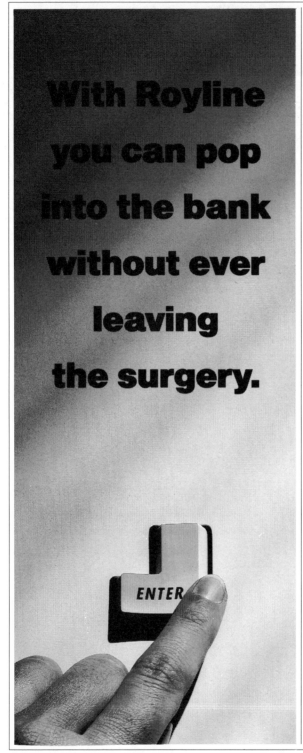

With Royline you can pop into the bank without ever leaving the surgery.

ENTER

We know how much work can be involved in running a surgery. Particularly with the introduction of the new contract.

It has meant an increase in general administration and the need for tighter financial control all round.

Fortunately, you can greatly ease your workload at the press of a button. With Royline. An easy to use, computer-based banking service from The Royal Bank of Scotland which gives you immediate access to your business and personal accounts.

With Royline you can transfer money into any account with any UK bank – without having to write out cheques or fill in forms. And receive up to date information on all incoming transactions (so you can see if the F.H.S.A./Health Board Payment has arrived), without leaving the surgery.

All you need is an IBM compatible personal computer – if you haven't already got one, a Government Grant may be available.

We'll do the rest. Including installation of the Royline software package and full training for you and your staff. Completely free of charge.

To find out more about Royline and our other services for GPs phone free on 0800 121 121.

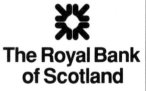

The Royal Bank of Scotland

THERE IS A DIFFERENCE

Organising Practice Finances

John Dean

There can be few if any systems of payment as complex and confusing as those for general practitioners in the NHS. As independent contractors, they are not paid a salary but derive their income from such sources as they generate through their commitment, efficiency and successful management of the practice.

Most GPs, of course, earn the bulk of their income from the NHS, but can also receive earnings from other sources, and many practices prosper as a result.

Since the introduction of the new GP contract in 1990 and the start of GP Fundholding in 1991, the body which most practices deal with on a regular basis is the family health service authority (FHSA), which is responsible for organising GP finances immediately above practice level. A further control on GPs' finance is 'cash limiting', which limits funds which FHSAs have at their disposal and which they can pass on to practices. This can lead to restrictions on surgery development or ancillary staff refunds.

Financial efficiency

It is one of the minor mysteries of medical practice why some GPs earn much more than others. The biggest single determinant is the efficiency of the practice. A practice may do well medically, be well thought of by its patients and be clinically efficient, yet be earning a low income. Other factors are the size of the patient list and the control of expenses.

Financial efficiency can encompass several factors, notably:

- a workable and practical in-house accounting system;

- adequate staffing levels;

- maximising of income levels;

- efficient claiming of refunds;

- computerisation;

- a general commitment to good management and financial efficiency by all the partners.

Against these may be set lifestyle aspirations that GPs and practice staff have. A practice may, for instance, choose to minimise night visits by employing costly deputising services. That is their privilege, so long as the practice is run properly and the contract fulfilled, but they must accept that it may lower their earnings.

The practice manager's role

In all this the practice manager is essential. It is she or he on whom the partners will depend for the efficient running of the business. Ideally, the practice manager will be in charge of the entire financial and management function – answerable to the partners to some degree but, within the guidelines of accepted practice policy, able to control his or her own work and delegate to staff. The best analogy is with the commercial world, where a business would largely be run by a company secretary. It is this role which more precisely defines that of the practice manager.

Management in general practice now offers an attractive career. In larger partnerships, a manager may well be running a business with a turnover of more than £1 million, plus any income from a dispensing or fundholding practice.

Much of the practice manager's work involves organising the practice finances – making sure that cash flow is properly controlled, that the accounting system is accurate and up to date, that partners' drawings are paid out regularly and systematically, that the bank account is run responsibly and that there is proper budgeting.

The practice manager is responsible for staffing levels, ensuring that they are adequate and that full ancillary staff refunds are received from the FHSA. Both the practice manager and his or her staff should have proper contracts of employment, with salaries regularly reviewed and duties clearly set out. A management chart enables the line of responsibility and control to be clearly understood.

E M I S

EGTON MEDICAL INFORMATION SYSTEMS LIMITED

EMIS has been designed by Doctors for Doctors to offer the flexibility, scope and sophistication required of a truly valuable clinical management tool. Further, it offers a practical, user-friendly path to full practice computerisation.

The system is fast, easy to learn and use, requiring virtually no computer literacy as all the options are menu driven. Its functionality is highly tailorable with numerous user definable screens and databases. The template facility enables users to define a screen or series of screens which prompt for information in situations defined by the user. It works as a computerised checklist. Where strict management guidelines need to be followed the protocol system can be used. The EMIS protocol system is the equivalent of a virtual expert system shell. It is highly flexible and can be tailored to almost any use where management or clinical guidelines need to be followed. Fully integrated dispensing, fundholding, word processing, targeting, auditing and communications software completes the system.

The communications package incorporates the FHSA GP Links software that establishes electronic data interchange (EDI) links between G.Ps and F.H.S.As.

EMIS has also developed a clinical information and decision support system for medical practitioners. It can be used as a simple textbook to look up layered medical facts or as a powerful, interactive real-time decision support tool that relates its output to the problems of a particular patient. The knowledge base is primed with concise summaries of disease reproduced from the Oxford Handbooks of Medicine.

Income generation

Most of the practice's income comes from the NHS in fees, allowances and direct refunds for a number of items.

The essential guide to the practice fees and allowances due to GPs is set out in the Red Book, which is updated three or four times a year. It is essential to have one that is up to date, and the practice manager, and at least one doctor, should be reasonably familiar with its contents. More complete details and updated information on current rates of fees and allowances can be obtained from the main medical journals such as *Medeconomics*, *Financial Pulse* and *Money Pulse*.

Following recent major changes in the GP contract, the main sources of practice income are:

- Practice allowances
    Basic practice allowance;
    Seniority awards;
    Postgraduate Education Allowance.

- Capitation payments
    Capitation fees (three age bands);
    Deprivation payments;
    Registration fees;
    Child health surveillance;
    Target payments:
       Childhood immunisation;
       Pre-school boosters;
       Cervical cytology.

- Sessional fees
    Health promotion (amended from 1 July 1993);
    Minor surgery payments;
    Student teaching fees.

Each of these headings of income has its own rules, which must be clearly understood. Every practice must be aware of its proper entitlement and ensure that claims are made efficiently.

Although fees and allowances are usually paid quarterly, practices should ensure that they receive monthly payments on account. These normally represent a third of the fees and allowances which can reasonably be forecast.

Item of service fees

Perhaps the biggest single factor in determining a practice's NHS income is the efficiency with which item of service fees are claimed. The average return on these represents 16 per cent of total fees and allowances. In a large practice, these can come to a substantial sum, and the efficiency with which they are claimed determines the level of practice income.

Item of service fees include night visit fees, temporary residents, contraceptive services, emergency treatment, maternity medical services and vaccinations.

Success in claiming these fees is a three tier exercise involving the doctor who, having seen a patient who qualifies for an item of service fee, completes the appropriate form, and the practice manager (or to whomever the work is delegated), who processes the claim, and then on receiving the fee checks it against practice records. This latter is important because FHSAs can make mistakes.

Outside work

The typical general practice will not, however, confine its activity to NHS patients. Many will derive an income from non-NHS sources or from other sources within the health service such as clinical assistants at local hospitals. Also, most practices will receive fees for insurance reports and medical examinations. Income from cremation fees, too, must be paid into practice funds and properly recorded.

Some practices will pick up further income from work at local hospitals, nursing homes, schools and so on. Many practices, especially in prosperous areas, may earn private patient fees. A further source of fees can be work as a medical officer to a company or business house. If possible, this should be on a retainer basis, so that this income comes in regularly.

In addition, practices will receive a steady stream of income from sundry cash fees from patients for signing certificates, passport applications and the like. Again it is essential that these are all paid into practice funds and recorded for tax purposes. Otherwise, the practice may be subjected to an Inland Revenue enquiry, which is best avoided.

One problem which particularly affects partnerships is deciding whether fees from non-NHS sources are paid into practice funds or retained by the individual doctors. This depends on the policy of the partnership, but those with a tradition of financial discipline ensure that all fees from medical sources are paid into practice funds and divided accordingly. This policy is not only more equitable but tends to minimise disputes.

A practice which enjoys an unusually high level of fees from non-NHS sources, 10 per cent or more of total income, runs the danger of suffering abatement of its direct refunds. This seldom happens and can be avoided with sound advice.

Direct refunds

A salient feature of the GP's remuneration package is an entitlement to direct refunds for certain items of expenditure, chiefly:

Surgery: Rent (leased surgeries)
               Notional or cost rent allowances (owner-occupied surgeries)
               Rates
               Refuse collection charges
Staffing: Ancillary staff
               Staff salaries (70 per cent or cash limit)
               National Insurance contributions (100 per cent or cash limit)
               Staff training costs (normally 70 per cent)
Trainees' salaries
Dispensing costs.

Again, these refunds must be claimed on a systematic basis. It is not unusual for practices to delay reclaiming their rates, for instance, and that can reduce the practice's profits.

'Grossing-up'

In addition to direct refunds, practices receive a theoretical indirect reimbursement of all other expenses, calculated by averaging expenses out among all GPs in the country on the basis of a selection of accounts submitted to the Inland Revenue.

It follows that it is to the advantage of all that these refunded expenses are maximised by showing them on both sides of the annual practice accounts. This ensures that the expenses should accurately reflect the costs of running the practice. But such 'netting out' still occurs surprisingly often, costing GPs as a whole thousands of pounds a year in unrecorded, and hence unreimbursed, expenses.

Cost economy

Just as maximising income is essential, so is controlling costs. Practices must constantly seek to reduce expenses. In 1993/94, GPs' gross remuneration increases are limited to only 3.7 per cent but it will be very hard for practices to keep their increased spending down to the same extent. Many find that expenses rise by 20 per cent a year. That discrepancy could mean a severe drop in net income for a practice. So how can practices control or even reduce these costs?

One major item for many practices is locum fees and relief services. Paying deputising services for night and weekend cover is expensive and because it attracts a reduced night visit fee, is doubly disadvantageous. Again, this depends on the quality of life members of the practice wish to enjoy. But they must accept that deputising fees will prevent profits from being maximised, especially at a time of severe income restraint.

Locum fees are another expense which gets out of hand in many practices. Is it really necessary to engage a locum when a partner is sick or on holiday? Can the other partners not cover for him or her?

Many practices spend too much on telephones. Try to make sure that only practice calls are made and encourage staff to cut down on private ones, or put a bar on other than local calls. Try to ensure that outward calls are made after 1 pm. A free itemised bill will highlight unusually costly calls. Calls may be shorter if the caller has to stand up!

Use stationery sensibly. Are separate letter headings and billheads for each partner necessary, for instance? Make all purchases in bulk, and seek discounts from wholesalers rather than using local stationers. Whenever possible use second class post. There will be urgent items but most letters do not have to arrive the next day.

In short, strict budgeting procedures should be applied to all expenditure.

Successful budgeting

All successful businesses, general practices among them, must have a strict expenditure budget. Sadly, all too many practices allow spending to get out of control, with no checks or any proper authorisation of payments.

For cheques over a certain level, say £50, signatures of more than one partner are advisable. Expenditure over say, £500, depending on the size of the practice, should be authorised by a partners' meeting. If a practice manager controls this budget, he or she should have some authority as a cheque signatory.

At the start of each accounting year, a budget should be drawn up on a monthly basis, allocating expenditure when it falls due. This should be built into a full budgeting procedure for the year in order to forecast income and profit. To a large extent, the budget will use analyses from previous years derived from annual accounts. Forecasts of such routine items as staff salaries, lighting and heating, telephone costs, rates, maintenance charges and the like are relatively easy to make.

Try to prepare the budget on a cumulative basis, updating it each month as the actual figures become available. Remember to keep the original forecast: this will show where variations have occurred.

Build a contingency reserve for unexpected items into the budget. For instance, if the roof needs repair at a cost of thousands, it might not have been possible to forecast but it could come out of this contingency fund.

Using statistics

One useful aspect of GP finance is that there is no lack of statistics against which the performance of a particular practice can be compared. For instance, the accepted percentages of income from NHS fees and allowance are:

Practice allowances	17
Capitation	63
Item of service fees	16
Sessional fees	4
Total	100

Income from practice allowances and capitation fees largely depends on factors outside the practice's control. The level of capitation fees, as with practice allowances, is fixed by the Government and the practice must therefore look to both sessional and item of service fees for extra income.

A comparison of practice results should be prepared each year, taking accrued items into account and comparing them with national averages. This will tell a great deal about the performance of the practice.

Another valuable statistic concerns item of service fees. It is this more than anything which affects the level of GPs' income and it in turn is affected by the efficiency with which work is done and claims pursued. For the 1991/92 year, the last full year for which information is available, the average item of service fees per patient in England and Wales was:

	£
Night visits	1.20
Temporary residents	0.33
Contraceptive services	0.87
Emergency treatment	0.04
Maternity medical service	1.37
Vaccinations	0.49
Total	4.30

It is important that practices analyse their item of service fees and compare them with these averages, which are a valuable tool for assessing the efficiency with which claims are processed.

This return largely depends on where the practice is. For instance, a practice in a holiday resort may well find that its income from temporary resident fees is well above average, whereas those in rural areas will have below average maternity fees. Further figures allow us to compare income generated from a practice, both gross and net, against the intended average remuneration. Gross intended income for a GP for the year ended 31 March 1993 was £59,977, while the net intended income was £40,010. For 1993/94, the corresponding figures are £62,305 gross and £40,113 net.

Business planning

All successful businesses plan ahead. The reasons for success are many and varied; there may be a successful product with a guaranteed sale, for instance, but nevertheless such a business will prosper even more with forward planning. Business planning has often saved businesses from going to the wall.

Such an outcome may be a little fanciful with regard to general practice, but even so most practices will benefit from forward planning. It will be able to plan its future, hopefully ensuring its continued success and enabling partners and staff to lead a more congenial lifestyle, and it will point to possible economies and efficient management procedures.

Most plans have been prepared under the Government's Enterprise Initiative Scheme, which has offered grants towards the cost of outside consultants who prepare the plan.

Unfortunately, these grants have been cut recently. Nevertheless, while the facility exists, practices should make use of it. It is likely that the Enterprise Initiative Scheme will end from 31 March 1994, so practices should take steps to do so as soon as possible. This work is probably best done by an outside consultant, who can look at the project objectively. Practices which have prepared their own plans have not been as successful. The consultant must, of course, have experience of both medical practice and business procedures.

The cost is a matter for negotiation between the practice, the consultant and the Department of Trade and Industry, which fixes consultants' fees. These can run from £200 to £450 a day. A practice which obtains a full DTI grant will, after tax relief, pay no more than about £100 a year per partner over five years, an acceptable price for the security of a professionally prepared plan.

Controlling Practice Finances

John Dean

Of the 32,000 GPs in the United Kingdom, about 26,000 practice in groups or partnerships, in which they pool profits and divide them in agreed ratios.

The classic definition of a business partnership is 'two or more people working together with a view for profit'; a more light-hearted definition has been that a partnership is the most intimate form of association outside marriage. This is not far from the truth, particularly in general practices, where doctors work closely together and must have common aims, regular meetings to set practice policy and an efficient management system.

Accounts

The practice will draw its accounts up to an agreed date, normally for a 12 month period, whatever changes may have occurred during the preceding year. As a rule, the best accounting date for practices is 30 June. That is the earliest quarter end within the tax year, thus allowing tax on realised profits to be paid at a later date than it would have been otherwise.

Each partner should know the amount of his or her capital contribution and how his or her monthly drawings are calculated and the profits shared. The accounts should set these details out in clear, precise terms so that equity is maintained.

Practice accounts are necessary for many reasons: to agree the annual tax liability, as possible evidence of financial rectitude when loans are negotiated; to maintain equity between partners, and to aid the recruitment of new partners. Accounts are an essential management tool, highlighting both possible economies and sources of new income.

It is likely that a partnership deed will specify that accounts are to be prepared and signed by the partners. To ensure that this is done systematically at minimum cost, a sound in-house accounting system is essential. Some practices now have computerised accounting packages but most practices continue to use manual bookkeeping systems, perfectly acceptable as long as they are efficient and accurate. The practice accountant should always be asked to advise on a system before it is installed.

Petty cash

All practices will use cash for small items of expenditure, but should pay for as many items as possible by cheque. The less cash that is kept in the surgery, the greater the security.

Petty cash records should be kept in a cash book and all expenses should have a receipt. Most practices will receive cash from patients, for certificates and the like, and this should be accounted for separately and paid into the bank without deduction. Keeping cash from patients and cash for defraying small expenses separate avoids confusion.

The practice cash book

In a manual bookkeeping system, the major accounting requirement is for an analysis cash book, written up regularly so that it is possible at any date to see the total accumulated expenditure under each heading in a given period. The book should be balanced monthly and reconciled with the bank account, usually at the end of the month or accounting year. The balances on the bank statements and in the cash book are likely to differ because cheques take at least three days to clear, so a reconciliation statement should take that into account.

A written-up cash book correctly balanced and reconciled is the biggest single determinant of how much work the accountant must do, and can therefore help to reduce accountancy costs. The cash book may be written up by the practice manager or delegated to a bookkeeper or another member of staff.

Partnership capital

All businesses must run on capital. In a professional partnership, the business is owned by the partners and it is they who contribute that capital. As a very general rule, the higher the capital, the higher the

The Yorkshire Clinic

Our long established reputation for quality patient care is enhanced by the completion of our £6 million development programme providing 72 beds with superb hotel services for the benefit of both patients and visitors.

Facilities now include four operating theatres, a Day Case Unit with its own theatre and recovery suite, a new Health Screening Clinic, enlarged Physiotherapy, Pathology and X-Ray Departments, Ultrasound Scanning, Cardiac and Vascular Catheterisation and Magnetic Resonance Imaging (MRI). In addition our programme of PGEA accredited seminars and training courses enables us to respond to the needs of your Practice.

All these developments mean even higher standards of medical treatment and patient care for our local community.

earnings. The capital in a typical medical practice consists of property, fixed assets and working capital. The surgery's total capital represents the investment of the partners in the equity, which is the balance remaining after deduction of all outstanding loans. If, for instance, a surgery has a current valuation of £500,000 but a mortgage secured on it of £400,000, this leaves a balance of equity of £100,000. If the building is owned equally by five partners, each thus has an investment of £20,000 in the equity.

In most medical practices, however, the surgery is owned by the partners in different proportions to those in which they share the profits. Some of the partners, for instance, may be partly retired doctors who have sold their shares in the building, or partners working their way to parity, or part-time doctors who do not want to be involved in surgery ownership. In such cases, the partners who own the building will be recompensed by an equivalent share in the notional or cost rent allowance. Likewise, they will be responsible for servicing any surgery loans.

The fixed asset capital normally represents the investment of the partners in non-surgery assets such as computers, furniture and fittings, medical equipment and the like. In a modern medical practice, possibly highly computerised, this can run into tens of thousands of pounds.

It is usual for the partners to own this capital in the same proportions as those in which they share the profits. The working capital of the practice is represented by the net current assets – typically, any sundry debts, cash at bank, less the amount owed to outstanding creditors. That is the money the practice needs to run on a day-to-day basis without going into the red.

A refinement of this is to combine fixed asset and working capital in a form of fixed practice capital, so that each partner knows their required contribution exactly. This helps to smooth financial transactions on partnership changes and means that when the accounts are completed each year, the partners can see that the balances on their current accounts represent undrawn profits which can be paid to them.

It is essential in all practices that the partners understand the principle of capital, how they contribute it, how they can most efficiently borrow the money, if necessary, and how it can best be organised for tax purposes.

Sharing the profits

As we have seen, most doctors practice as members of partnerships, sharing profits in agreed ratios. It is essential that these are known, that they are set down properly in the partnership deed and that on production of the annual accounts the practice manager can see that the profit has been divided correctly.

It is common, but by no means universal, for a young partner joining a practice to do so for a probationary period during which he or she will earn a fixed share or a percentage. This both encourages the partner to increase the profits of the practice, in which he or she will have a share, while giving an element of security with a minimum level of income.

In many cases, practices will recruit doctors on a 'fixed share basis', often incorrectly referred to as a 'salaried partnership', the 'fixed share partner' being paid a fixed sum rather than a percentage. Despite this, he or she is a partner in every sense. This doctor should have a share in the running and management of the practice, be shown as a partner in the annual practice accounts and generally be seen to act as a full partner. Failure to do this means that the practice runs the risk of losing its basic practice allowance, which is paid only to principals in general medical practice.

Calculation of drawings

Another point of controversy in practices is the way in which drawings are paid to individual practitioners.

It should be emphasised that the payments they receive at the end of each month are not 'salary', but drawings. As such, they are payments on account of eventual profits, which cannot be quantified exactly until the end of each financial year. Such drawings may take all kinds of variations between the partners into account, such as differing rates of seniority, income tax, national insurance, postgraduate education allowance and added years of superannuation. As a result, it is unlikely that in a practice with equal partners, their drawings will be equal. Some may be buying added years, or have higher tax liabilities than their colleagues.

It is also a fact of life that drawings can go down as well as up. When, for some innocent reasons, drawings have been overpaid to a partner, it may be preferable to repay by reducing future drawings rather than paying a lump sum. And, of course, profits can go down as well as up.

There are many ways of calculating drawings. Perhaps the simplest is for them to be paid out monthly in line with profit-sharing ratios. In a complex partnership – as most GP partnerships are – it is inevitable that when accounts are drawn up, there will be differences in the partners' current accounts which will largely reflect the accuracy with which periodic drawings have been calculated.

More sophisticated systems can involve the preparation of 'equalised drawings', whereby a projection of future profits is taken, all known adjustments made and one-twelfth of their net disposable income paid to the partners at the end of each month. This system is attractive to many practice members, although it can only be as accurate as the original estimates used.

Income tax

Although taxation is a fact of life, that is not to say that it cannot be organised to the best advantage of a practice. Because GPs are self-employed, they have a great deal of scope to organise their affairs to minimise their tax liability.

It is often proposed that practices spend money to save tax, but that is false economy. It may well reduce tax liability but the whole purpose of the exercise is to save money through saving tax. If, for instance, a practice spends money on redecorating the surgery or buying a new car when it is unnecessary, the cost will indeed be fully allowed for tax purposes but even on a 40 per cent tax rate, the practice will still be 60 per cent out of pocket.

Most doctors are taxable under either Schedule D or Schedule E. Schedule E, or PAYE tax, is paid by most people who are employees. Its main feature is that, as it is taken from wages or salaries at the time and place of payment, the employee has little control over the amount deducted. In addition, the rules for claiming tax relief on expenses are stringent.

GPs, however, are self-employed people and pay tax under Schedule D, a rather different prospect. Tax is not deducted at source but is usually paid in two instalments on 1 January and 1 July each year. The Inland Revenue is more relaxed about claiming practice expenses. GPs are assessed on the preceding year, which means that taxable profits are assessed in a single tax year on the basis of profits generated in the previous accounting year. For example, if a practice makes its accounts up to 30 June, those for the year to 30 June 1993 will form the basis of assessment for tax in the assessment year 1994/95, and tax will be payable on 1 January and 1 July 1995, up to two years after the money has been earned. This greatly benefits cash flow and with good advice can be used to the best advantage of the practice. However, this is about to change (see Chapter 3.4). But that does not mean that GPs will no longer benefit from the system. Within the next year or so, practices should be discussing with their professional advisers how their finances can be organised to derive as much benefit as they can from changes in the rules.

Doctors in partnership are assessed on the same basis, except that their profits for taxation purposes are divided on the basis of profit-sharing ratios in the year of assessment rather than those in the period during which they were earned, which may be different. GPs can also, of course, obtain relief for personal expenses, where these are not paid out of practice funds.

National insurance

All GPs under the age of 65 (60 for women) pay national insurance, possibly in Classes 2 and 4. Class 2 national insurance represents a weekly amount (1993/94: £5.55), normally paid either by direct debit or quarterly. Class 4 contributions (1993/94 maximum £976.50) are paid by an addition to the half-yearly income tax demand. Doctors who have part-time hospital appointments may also have to make contributions under Class 1. There is, however, a maximum payment under all classes each year and steps must be taken to see that doctors apply, if necessary, for deferment of Classes 2 and 4 or, in the absence of this, claim refunds of contributions overpaid after the end of each year.

Tax reserves

It is strongly recommended that all partnerships set aside funds regularly to provide for future tax liabilities. This has a number of benefits. Partnership tax at present is assessed on the practice as a whole, so if a partner has, for instance, left the practice or has become bankrupt and cannot pay his share of this liability, it falls back on the other partners. That can be avoided by setting sums aside, either physically or within the accounts, which will ensure that there are funds to meet such liabilities.

Insurance

All practices should insure against fire, burglary, third party risks and other items. This may well be done under some form of comprehensive traders policy. Professional indemnity will be covered by one of the recognised defence organisations.

Doctors often seek to insure against sickness and to cover the cost of locums by taking out permanent health insurance policies. That is right and prudent, but premiums are not allowable for tax purposes. In the event of a claim, however, the benefit will not be taxable either for a period of one year.

Similarly, GPs may wish to take out policies for private medical insurance. Substantial discounts can be obtained if the practice forms a group scheme.

The practice accountant

A practice should be able to rely on its accountant to deal efficiently with the accountancy and taxation affairs both of the practice and the partners and to give advice on all kinds of financial problems which may affect the practice, including cost rent schemes, pension and retirement planning and management.

It is a relationship which at its best can be rewarding to both sides but at worst can degenerate into distrust and even hostility, with the practice feeling the accountant is not acting in its best interests, does not understand how the system works, is not giving good advice and is possibly overcharging. This may happen but sadly some practices never really find what they are looking for – which indeed, may be unobtainable. Practices which are constantly changing accountants may find the root of their problem in their own practice rather than outside it.

What qualities should a practice look for in an accountant and how should they judge if he is looking after their best interests? Points to consider, in order of importance, are:

1   Is he or she a specialist?
2   Is he or she efficient?
3   Fee levels; and
4   Location.

Perhaps above all, the accountant should be a specialist in general practice finance. There is little point in engaging an accountant who, although highly qualified, experienced and well versed in other fields, has never dealt with general practices. It may well cost the practice a lot of money to fund his or her learning curve. Does he or she have a copy of the Red Book and keep it up to date?

Whether or not the accountant is a specialist, he or she should also be able to demonstrate a level of efficiency and urgency. Will letters be answered quickly? If he or she is away, can somebody else deal with the work? Are telephone calls returned reasonably promptly? Can someone in the office give detailed advice, over the telephone if necessary?

Partnerships invariably find that matters work much more easily if the same accountant deals with the personal affairs of the individual partners as well as those of the practice itself. This minimises communications and contacts, saving time and costs.

The accountant should, of course, prepare the annual practice accounts and get them agreed by the Inland Revenue. In addition, he or she may be asked to give one-off specialist advice from time to time.

When acting for individual partners, duties will mainly consist of preparing and agreeing their annual income tax returns and expense claims, agreeing assessment notices, approving demands for payment, submitting appeals and the like. In addition, he or she is likely to become involved in pensions and estate planning, as well as advising on a whole range of personal matters.

Fees are always a matter of concern between general practices and their accountants. This is largely within the control of the practice itself. Fees are much less if the practice manager presents the accountant with a full set of annual records, fully balanced and reconciled. Practices should, however, obtain an annual quotation of likely costs and see that this is adhered to.

GP Fundholding

Jackie Roberts

Fundholding was first proposed in the Government's White Paper, *Working for Patients*, in January, 1989. It was subsequently enacted as the National Health Service and Community Care Act 1990.

Entry into the fundholding scheme enables the individual practice to manage a portion of the total funds for the region in order to purchase care for its own patients. The scheme offers the practice an opportunity to improve services for patients, bringing many treatments in-house and taking steps to reduce waiting times.

The fund is divided in the legislation into three components: hospital and community health services, prescribing costs and ancillary staff costs. Fundholders' budgets are presently set by most regional health authorities by reference to historical levels of activity and expenditure, although there is a move towards 'capitation based' funding. That would mean budgets being set according to the number of patients on the practice list, taking certain weighting factors into account rather than by reference to levels of known activity.

Eligibility criteria

Practices must satisfy a number of eligibility criteria to become fundholders:

1 there must be at least 7,000 patients on the practice list;
2 all members of the practice must agree to become fundholders and are bound by the actions of the others in this context;
3 if more than one partnership share a fund in order to satisfy the list size criterion, there must be an agreement to the effect that all members are bound by each other's actions in the context of fundholding; and

4   the practice must show that it can effectively manage a fund. This is intended to cover staffing arrangements, management structure and other practice resources, in particular a computer system which can handle a fundholding software package which conforms to the Department of Health's specification.

Once the practice has begun fundholding, the following additional requirements must be fulfilled to maintain continuing recognition as a fundholding practice:

1   a separate fundholding bank account is maintained, into which is paid any cash received in respect of the staffing budget or reimbursement of fund savings expenditure (see below);
2   the practice must submit monthly accounts to the responsible family health service authority (FHSA) by the end of each month in respect of transactions relating to the previous month. These accounts include an income and expenditure account and a balance sheet in respect of the fundholding side of the practice;
3   annual accounts must be submitted to the responsible FHSA within six weeks of the end of the financial year (31 March).

Other, fairly complex regulations govern the purchasing and provision of services for patients of the fundholding practice by members of the practice from bodies in which those members have an interest. These should be reviewed carefully before the practice decides to proceed along those lines.

Management of fundholding

The preparatory year

In the year leading up to a practice becoming a fundholder (the preparatory year), the practice will normally be engaged in a data collection exercise, counting hospital referral statistics and information on the provision of community care on behalf of the practice. This information may be used to set the budget by applying the prices to be charged by the practice's usual provider units in the fundholding year. Although it is strictly necessary only to collect data on services currently covered by the fundholding scheme, many authorities consider that practices should collect all referral statistics, and over as long a period as possible. Although district nursing and health visiting are currently funded by reference to the number of whole time equivalent staff available to the practice, it is useful to collect data on the number of patients seen by these staff, and how their time is occupied. In this way, the practice can more effectively negotiate any required improvements to the level of service into their contracts with community units.

Where budgets for the hospital and community health element of the budget are set by reference to a capitation formula, the above referral statistics will prove invaluable to the practice in determining whether the level of the budget offer is sufficient to meet patients' needs.

Practices should be aware of one of the main drawbacks of setting the level of the fund on the basis of historical information: if a service has not been available to the practice in the past, it is likely that the practice will not be funded for that service in the future. It will therefore be necessary to 'vire' monies from other parts of the budget to provide that service for the patients.

It is now a requirement that all fundholding practices prepare a business plan, by the autumn of their preparatory year, which will incorporate an outline of where the practice intends to place its contracts for hospital and community care. The business plan provides a firm foundation for the classic management model: plan, monitor and control. The plan should be prepared in sufficient detail, including financial statements and forecasts, to be used as a tool with which to monitor progress towards stated objectives.

The prescribing budget is set by reference to prescribing patterns in the preparatory year, and is adjusted for known high cost patients on the practice list as well as for the regional average costs per prescribing unit. It is therefore necessary for the practice to be aware of any factors which may affect prescribing cost levels after it begins fundholding.

The portion of the budget relating to reimbursable staff costs is normally set by reference to the staffing levels in the practice during the preparatory year. In common with non-fundholding practices, the amount of money allotted to fundholders for their staff is subject to the FHSA cash limits. Practices will need to review staffing levels during this year to ensure the budget is enough to meet their needs. The staffing budget does not provide for the salaries of staff employed in the administration of fundholding; these costs should be reimbursed out of the management allowance (see below).

Fundholding years

Once the practice has accepted the initial budget offer and becomes a full fundholder, it has accepted responsibility for part of the regional health authority resources and for purchasing hospital and community care for its patients within the constraints of the allotted sum. The practice must therefore be prepared and equipped to manage these resources efficiently and effectively.

Audit and control

The fundholding accounts are subject to audit by the Audit Commission. An individual practice may be audited each year, although the auditors may at their discretion perform an in-depth audit only once every three years. The practice will therefore need to satisfy the auditors that there are sufficient internal controls to ensure the accuracy of the fundholding accounts and the proper and efficient use of the monies. This will entail:

- designation of specific responsibilities and duties to partners and staff, ensuring that duties are properly segregated and staff adequately supervised;

- the fundholding accounts should be regularly reviewed in order to monitor progress and anticipate problems before they arise;

- the fundholding records, including the computer system, should be kept secure from unauthorised access, and adequate back-ups retained;

- staff should be carefully recruited with reference to qualifications and skills, and the practice should take care that they are properly trained in their duties; and

- the accounts must be fully reconciled each month with other records kept within the practice and also by other parties with whom it has dealings, such as the FHSA, the bank and the provider units.

The fundholding process

The initial budget allotted to the practice is held by the FHSA, who act as paying agents on behalf of the practice. Any additions to the initial budget (further fund allocation) are similarly dealt with.

Hospital and community health services

Referrals are generated by members of the practice in the usual way and entered on the fundholding computer system. The practice should be notified by the provider unit when treatment has started, so that this in turn can be entered. This entry gives rise to the cost of the treatment being accumulated as expenditure. When the invoice is received, this too is entered on the system and marked for payment as appropriate. A remittance advice is then produced which acts as authority to the FHSA to pay the provider. Payment should then be made by the FHSA directly to the provider.

If a block type contract is in force, where a regular monthly payment is made regardless of the level of activity undertaken by the provider, the same process applies, the practice authorising payment and the health authority making the transfer of cash.

The practice is not liable for treatment costs of more than £5,000 in respect of an individual patient during a single financial year. These will initially be paid for by the practice, but will be reclaimed from the patient's district health authority (DHA) of residence. The practice should anticipate these costs arising and inform the DHA wherever possible.

Prescribing costs

A monthly statement of prescribing costs is sent to the practice by the Prescription Pricing Authority. The total costs for each month are entered in the accounts. The FHSA pays the chemists directly on behalf of the practice.

Staff costs

The reimbursable proportion of staff costs is calculated by the practice each month, and entered onto the system in the form of an invoice from the general practice. Cash is received from the FHSA each month into the fundholding bank account, either in response to a requisition sent by the practice or as an instalment of the staff budget. In either case, the practice may then transfer only the amount claimed as reimbursable staff costs to the practice bank account, any surplus monies remaining on the fundholding bank account.

District nursing and health visiting

Monthly invoices are entered in the accounts and paid in the same way as the block contract invoices discussed above. The costs of providing these services are not attributed to individual patients and the contracts used are therefore called 'non-attributable contracts'.

Savings

Savings made during the course of the year can be used to supplement other parts of the budget during the same financial year. Some FHSAs require the practice to obtain their approval for such virements. The practice should consider whether the savings will be available in the long term before re-allocating the monies to the provision of ongoing services.

At the year-end, any savings made (total funds allotted less total expenditure incurred), taking into account all budget elements, are available for the practice's future use for the benefit of their patients. Such savings must first be approved by the Audit Commission auditors, and the expenditure out of savings must be approved by the FHSA.

Management allowance

To help defray the costs incurred in managing the fund, a management allowance is available to reimburse related expenditure such as salaries, postage and stationery, training, consultancy fees and equipment purchases. The allowance available to practices in full fundholding years is £35,000 for 1993/94, £17,500 being available to practices in their preparatory year. (Joint fundholders would share an allowance of £20,000 in their preparatory year.) Practices in their preparatory year may claim locum fees in respect of time spent by partners of the practice on fundholding matters up to a level of £3,718 (1993/94), while in full fundholding years, locum fees may only be claimed in respect of external locums. The locum allowance is part of, not an addition to, the management allowance. The amount which may be claimed during a single year for equipment purchases is restricted to 50 per cent of the preparatory year or 25 per cent of the full year allowance.

Computer reimbursements

Potential and full fundholders are entitled to claim up to 75 per cent of computer hardware costs; fundholding software, maintenance and training are fully reimbursable.

Summary

It can be seen that fundholding requires considerable input from the practice. However, the benefits to be gained for patients and the increased choice and responsibility for GPs have already led some 1,200 practices to become fundholders up to the third wave, with no sign of an abatement of interest from the prospective fourth wave of practices.

Taxation and the GP

Angela Britton

Proposals to change significantly the way in which partnerships and sole traders are taxed will affect all GPs who practise as principals. For many years, using the preceding year as the basis of assessment has brought significant tax advantages to sole traders and partners, including doctors, who have enjoyed the benefits of paying tax on less than their current earnings.

The Inland Revenue was unhappy about this, feeling that the current system of personal taxation was administratively cumbersome and difficult to understand, discouraging prompt payment. This led to two consultative documents which proposed replacing the preceding year basis of assessment with self-assessment. In his spring 1993 Budget, the Chancellor confirmed that legislation to bring in the changes would be included in the autumn 1993 Finance Bill.

In this article I will outline the proposals and then address some planning opportunities which they suggest. I would emphasise that until the proposals become law, and we see the full transitional rules as well as the anti-avoidance provisions, no irrevocable action should be taken.

The proposals

The Inland Revenue has stated that the aim of the new system is to be simpler, fairer and more straightforward, allowing the taxpayer greater control, reducing dealings with the tax authorities and lowering administration costs. The proposals will take effect from 6 April 1996 with 1996/97 a transition year and the new basis taking effect fully from 1997/98 onwards.

All income will be taxed on a current year basis and for sole traders and partnerships there are strong indications that the proposals will be as outlined in the second of the two consultative documents. Tax will be charged on the profits of the accounting period ending in the year of assessment.

For a practice with a 30 June year end the assessments will be:

1995/96	Year to 30 June 1994
1996/97	12/24 × 24 months to 30 June 1996
1997/98	Year to 30 June 1997

Half of the profits for the 24 months to 30 June 1996 will therefore not be taxed.

For partnerships, assessments will be on the individual partners (not the firm as now). This will cause major difficulties for large partnerships where the allocation of a payment to the partnership as a whole has allowed under and overpayments to be matched between partners without penal interest charges. That will no longer be possible. However, for most doctors' partnerships it should be possible to work out accurately the individual doctor's liabilities by the time the tax is payable. As the allocation of profits for tax will now be in the same ratio as when the profits are earned, this calculation should be easier to make. Changes in partnerships will no longer be deemed a cessation.

Choice of year end

Although any year end is possible, it is likely to prove beneficial for practices to change their accounting date to 31 March by 31 March 1997 at the latest. Under the proposed legislation, if a doctor retired on 30 June 1998, for example, he would pay tax for 1998/99 on a full year's profits, despite having left after only three months of the tax year. This is the Revenue's way of forcing a 31 March year end on all taxpayers. Whenever a firm changes its accounting date from 30 April to 31 March, the effect is that 11 of the 35 months to the new 31 March year end do not form the basis of any assessment. In static partnerships (with static numbers of partners/patients), profits are likely to rise, so a change in 1997 will give the maximum benefit. If, however, profits are likely to drop because the loss of a partner or patients or any excessive one-off expenditure, it would be sensible to ask your accountant to consider a change earlier.

Planning for the changes

Legitimate maximisation of profits in the transitional period will reduce the overall tax charge. For example:

Table 3.4.1

		Taxable profits £	Adjusted taxable profits £
Year to 30 June	1994	200	175
	1995	250	275
	1996	275	300
	1997	300	275
		£1,025	£1,025

Table 3.4.2

	Profits assessed	
	before adjustment £	after adjustment £
1995/96	200	175
1996/97	262	287
1997/98	300	275
	£762	£737

Maximisation of profit in the transitional period is more difficult for doctors than for some other businesses because of the predictability of their income, but it may be that certain expenditure can be brought forward or delayed.

A major area where doctors can save tax is on loans. Tax relief on interest paid by partners on personal loans is allowable in the actual tax year in which it is paid. Partnership loan interest is charged in the accounts, so half the relief for interest paid in the transitional period will be lost. If the partnership has existing loans or overdrafts, these should be replaced by additional partnership capital subscribed out of the partners' personal borrowings. Care needs to be taken where capital is recycled and you should take professional advice to ensure you do not lose relief on any interest on existing personal loans.

Similarly, capital allowances are given for the year of assessment, whereas lease costs are charged in the accounts. The advice here, therefore, is to buy assets rather than lease them.

Payment of tax

Under the new system tax will be paid in 3 instalments.

For 1997/98 tax year

1 January 1998	50% of 1996/97 liability
1 July 1998	50% of 1996/97 liability
1 January 1999	Balance of 1997/98 tax liability

For 1998/99 tax year

1 January 1999	50% of 1997/98 liability and so on

It is likely that 1996/97 tax will follow the new rules, so 1 January 1998 will be the first year when increased tax will be payable. For example:

Balance of 1996/97 liability (ie excess over 1995/96)
50%   of 1996/97 liability

There will be no payment in the first year of a new business. Payment will be made on all income less any tax already paid, such as PAYE or tax on dividends. No interim payments will be required if most income is already taxed at source, so Schedule E tax payers will usually have to make a payment only on 1 January following the year of assessment on higher rate tax on dividends etc. Interim payments will also be reduced if it can be shown that income has fallen.

Conclusion

The changes will certainly happen. They will accelerate tax where profits are rising. They should be simpler. At present, there are a number of planning opportunities, although we need to see the actual legislation, in particular the transitional rules and any anti-avoidance legislation. Doctors are therefore advised to review their affairs with their accountants after the autumn 1993 Finance Bill to ensure they organise their affairs to obtain maximum benefits from the proposals.

Part Four

Patient Care

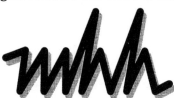

Community Nursing Services

Lynn Young

The best general practices have several different community nurses attached to them to provide a comprehensive, well-coordinated primary health care team for the practice population. Because general practices vary so much, the number and type of community nurses working with GPs also vary greatly from area to area. There have been examples of fine primary health care in action for many years, but unfortunately there are still practices in which there is little teamwork between GPs and community nurses – so much so that in some cases professionals working for the same practice population do not even know each other's names!

However, the 1990 NHS and Community Care Act has highlighted the need for better primary health care. As a result, there is now a greater drive and incentive for GPs and community nurses to work together and decide how best to deliver health care. The new GP contract brought rapid expansion in the number of practice nurses employed by GPs throughout the country. This caused much confusion at the time but things settled down in time for yet more change following the new health promotion banding system which started in July, 1993.

Although practice nurses often work closely with their community nurse colleagues, they have one fundamental difference. Practice nurses are employed by GPs but community nurses work for the district health authority community unit or community trust. As the 1990 reforms take an increasing grip on the NHS, almost all community nurses will soon be employed by trusts. So, while it is imperative for them to work in close cooperation with practice nurses, they have different employers and, very often, different conditions of work.

Primary health care teams, too, differ from practice to practice, some being bigger and more complicated than others. A fairly typical

WEIGHT WATCHERS

As a General Practitioner, referral of your patients to specialists is common practice and vital if you are to fulfil your professional responsibility by giving them the best possible service.

There are opthalmologists, ear nose and throat specialists, paediatricians, (obstetricians), dermatologists, physiotherapists, psychologists . . .

But who do you refer your patients to if they are overweight? Do you have time to devise a specially tailored diet suitable for their individual requirements? Does your patient really need to make an appointment with a dietician, if they don't have a serious eating disorder, but just need to improve their eating habits?

There is an organisation you can recommend with complete confidence, without compromising your patient's individual needs.

Weight Watchers, The UK's leading weight loss organisation, works hand in hand with the medical profession to ensure a safe, sensible and nutritionally sound Programme for their Members.

The Weight Watchers Programme is constantly updated with the advice and assistanc of leading nutritionists and medical experts and is fully in line with Government guidelines on nutrition and health, including the 1991 COMA report and the 1992 "Health of the Nation" White Paper.

The Weight Watchers Food Plan consists of **REAL** food, suitable for both Weight Watchers Members and their families, and it includes the required daily intake of vitamins, minerals, proteins and carbohydrates.

So comprehensive is the Weight Watchers Programme, it is far more than "just a diet", it's a way of life that teaches Members to **re-educate** their eating habits and change the way they think about food.

From January 1993, Weight Watchers will be offering people their best Programme ever! For the first time, the recently devised **"Quick and Simple"** Programme, encourages Members to choose their own Goal Weight. At the start of their weight loss Members select a target weight that suits them in consultation with you, their GP and our trained Meeting Leader. However, Members cannot set their target weight below the Weight Watchers recommended Goal Weight range.

As an unbending rule, Weight Watchers maintains scrupulous criteria for Membership. If an individual shows any signs of an eating disorder such as Anorexia Nervosa of Bulimia, Weight Watchers Meeting Leaders will immediately ask them to speak to you or to a specialist organisation.

Children below the age of 10 are not allowed to join Weight Watchers. Children between the ages of 10 and 16 **MUST** have their parent's **and** as their GP, your approval. All Members **MUST** have at least 7lbs of weight to lose.

Over the last 25 years, Weight Watchers has helped millions of people in the UK to lose weight. For your patients, there is no better way to improve their waistline and improve their health.

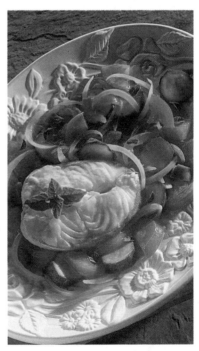

team will comprise GPs, a practice nurse, a health visitor, a district nurse, a community psychiatric nurse, a community mental handicap nurse and a school nurse. Some primary health care teams include a social worker, a community pharmacist, a midwife and a family planning nurse.

The NHS is undergoing such major change at present that it is almost impossible at times to see where GPs and community nurses are heading. GP fundholding further complicates the picture, especially since 1 April, 1993, when fundholders acquired enhanced purchasing powers so that they could contract for community nursing services from NHS community units.

But whatever changes are politically imposed, it is still vital to improve primary health care. That will not happen unless the role of the community nurse is understood by GPs and those they employ, such as practice managers and receptionists. Both practice and community nurses can enjoy a meaningful working relationship which involves a pooling of skills and resources and brings high quality services.

The practice nurse

Practice nursing is a 'growth industry'. Almost 18,000 are currently employed by the nation's GPs. Since the 1990 legislation, their work has expanded considerably, and it is likely to grow further as health care becomes increasingly based in general practice rather than hospitals. Practice nurses not only provide nursing treatments, but also run chronic disease and health promotion clinics, as well as health screening sessions in many cases.

Practice nurses often run their own surgeries, performing many nursing tasks, such as immunisation and vaccination clinics, well-woman and well-man clinics, and diabetes and asthma sessions. They carry out treatments such as ear syringing, wound dressings and injections, and provide health education when appropriate. New activities include cervical smears, family planning, breast and vaginal examinations and programmes for preventing cardiovascular disease. Practice nurses are becoming more involved in health promotion work like smoking cessation and weight reduction as well as health and nursing problems such as wound care. Increasingly, practice nurses, with their community nursing colleagues, will be devoting time to activities which contribute towards meeting the targets set out in the *Health of the Nation* White Paper.

Practice nurses are committed to helping people improve their health and take responsibility for it. Nowadays, patients and their families will often choose to visit the practice nurse rather than the GP.

The district nurse

The district nurse is a registered nurse who has obtained a District Nurse Diploma at a college of higher education. He or she offers skilled nursing care to those who wish to be nursed at home rather than in hospital. The district nurse is professionally responsible and accountable for assessing the needs of the family and ensuring that people who need nursing receive a high quality of care. District nurses visit people in their own homes or those in residential care, giving expert care to those with acute, chronic or terminal illness. The Community Care Act will bring more community nurses into a care management role.

In addition, district nurses often work with their practice nurse colleagues in the GP's treatment room, running leg ulcer, diabetes, continence and stoma care clinics. They are often able to prevent the need for patients to go into hospital and can facilitate their safe and early discharge if they are admitted. They can administer intravenous therapy and other care which was previously done mainly by hospital nurses. By imparting some simple self-help skills, they can help patients and carers to become increasingly independent.

District nurses give people information on a wide range of topics, including local facilities and services and welfare benefits, and refer them to health and social care services when appropriate.

In the course of their work, district nurses are often teaching others, such as student nurses, medical students, social workers, hospital staff and GP trainees. They set up and run self-care groups, especially for the many patient carers in most practice populations.

Health visitors

Like district nurses, health visitors are registered nurses, but have completed a further 12 months' education. The focus of their work is to promote health and well-being and prevent illness and disease. They work particularly with young children and their parents, though many provide a service to the whole family or even the community at large in group sessions like play groups, post-natal depression groups and carers' support groups. Health visitors have the expertise to assist fundholders in their obligatory twice-yearly profiles of the health needs of their practice populations, so that services can be targeted to people in most need. Health visitors can share this information with their primary health care colleagues and help develop services accordingly.

They also carry out child health assessments, which include child development screening and early detection of abnormality. They can manage and supervise immunisation programmes for children in clinics and give opportunistic immunisations at home. Much of the health visitor's work is to do with parenting skills, teaching parents to cope with babies' sleeping and crying, toilet training, weaning and temper tantrums. Advice is given on breast feeding and all aspects of nutrition.

Some health visitors identify health problems and plan appropriate health education programmes in such matters as accident prevention, HIV and AIDS, alcohol and drug abuse, cervical screening, stopping smoking and family planning. Health visitors have knowledge of child protection issues and can prevent child abuse following the early detection of family stress. This work (often in cooperation with local social services) includes helping the rehabilitation of families and children who have been abused. Among other health visiting activities are the identification and treatment of common minor childhood ailments, such as nappy rash, thrush, diarrhoea, vomiting and chickenpox. Advice, health promotion and education are always on hand where there is a health visiting service.

Community psychiatric nurses

Community psychiatric nurses are registered mental health nurses, many of whom have completed post-registration courses which equip them to work in the community, alongside GPs. They can carry out assessments of mental health in a family or social context and offer a therapeutic and supportive service to people who suffer from many kinds of mental health problems – behaviour therapy, for instance, can be given for certain acute neurotic episodes such as obsessive compulsive phobias. Long-term care and support can be given to a whole family when one of its members suffers from acute or chronic psychotic illness, such as schizophrenia.

Community psychiatric nurses often offer services for people who are in distress rather than clinically ill, as in marital and relationship therapy, family therapy, stress management, sexual dysfunction therapy and genetic counselling. They can also set up rehabilitation programmes for substance abuse and are a valuable source of information on the management of violent and aggressive behaviour and all aspects of community mental health. Community psychiatric nurses are becoming increasingly involved in the integration of mentally ill people into the community and in doing so, work towards dispelling myths and allaying fears which many people have.

Community mental handicap nurses

Each general practice should have its named registered mental handicap nurses, but unfortunately not all do. However, as primary health care develops and more people with learning disabilities are discharged from residential care into the community, more mental handicap nurses should become part of the typical general practice team.

Their key skill is to assess patients' potential and, with the assistance of family and carers, help them to achieve the best possible quality of life. They aim to increase the self-esteem of their patients and to give support to family members. Often, by accessing a wide range of services, they can relieve the burdens borne by many carers.

Community mental handicap nurses increase people's potential through behaviour modification and occupational and play therapy. They are particularly good at managing violent and aggressive behaviour and help to integrate people with learning disabilities into the community. This aspect of their work will become increasingly important in the light of the Community Care Act. Other activities are similar to those of all community nurses, such as helping with carers' support groups, giving advice on welfare benefits and acting as a resource for student nurses, medical students and GP trainers.

The school nurse

School nurses are usually attached to specific schools as well as being members of the primary health care team. They aim to help reduce the level of children's health problems. Their traditional role is undergoing much change at present and many now describe themselves as occupational nurses for schoolchildren. Health promotion is an increasingly important aspect of school nursing and services are being directed towards children with special needs and particular health problems. School nurses are often responsible for managing immunisation and vaccination programmes; they conduct full health interviews and give health advice to students. They can give confidential help and advice on such diverse and sometimes sensitive subjects as acne, exam pressures and sexual health.

General practice staff should realise that current changes put community nurses under great strain. NHS structures are being dismantled and more people discharged from hospitals. There is no doubt that many community nurses are already overstretched. But they continue to endeavour to meet the health needs of their patients and remain at the forefront of change, learning new skills and knowledge to meet growing, and increasingly complex, demands. Together, community nurses and GPs will develop a truly comprehensive primary health care system which will enhance the health of their practice populations in the 1990s and beyond.

Prescribing and Formulary

David Clegg

The Prescription and Pricing Authority (PPA), based in Newcastle-upon-Tyne, calculates and categorises each practice's prescribing costs and provides that information to the practice. Prescribing Analyses and Costs (PACT) reports give a three-level analysis every three months.

Level 1 is a simple quarterly analysis of a practice's prescribing. It compares its costs and its volume of prescribing with the average for practices of the same size and structure in the same family health services authority (FHSA). On the first page, bar charts show the comparison for net ingredient cost (NIC), volume or number of items prescribed, and cost per item. Usually, the more items prescribed (volume), the lower the cost per item, but the final test of prescribing economy is the NIC.

The second and third pages show the cost under six chapter headings of the British National Formulary (BNF): cardiovascular system, musculo-skeletal and joint diseases, gastrointestinal system, central nervous system, and endocrine system (the latter introduced in 1993 to replace infections). These chapters have been chosen because they contain the most costly drugs.

The last page shows information for the individual GP as well as for the practice. This includes the number of items that have been prescribed generically, the number of patients on the practice list and the number of prescribing units (PUs). Under a system known as Astro PUs, patients are graded by age and sex to reflect their likely usage of drugs.

Level 2 draws attention to prescribing costs and shows where they are highest in the six BNF chapters, listing the costliest drugs in each section of the chapters. Level 2 is sent automatically to any practice which is 25 per cent above the local average or which is 75 per cent over in any individual chapter, but as Level 2 is useful for looking at major items of expense, a practice may obtain this information even if it has not exceeded these limits.

Level 3 may be requested by an individual or a practice. If, in a training practice, a trainee's FP 10 form has been endorsed with a 'D', the trainee's Level 3 report comes automatically.

The first three pages of the Level 3 report repeat those of Level 2. On the following pages, the items are divided into 21 chapters corresponding with the chapters in the BNF. The total number of items, the total cost, the items and cost per 1,000 patients and per 1,000 PUs, are all given for each therapeutic category. Every item dispensed during the quarter is then listed, with the amount prescribed and its cost. The full Level 3 report for a practice may run to more than 100 pages. It is useful for learning and audit, and for starting a practice formulary. It is the acid test of a practice's prescribing.

Indicative prescribing amounts

Indicative Prescribing Amounts (IPAs) are the sums assigned to all practices within which they should seek to keep their prescribing costs. They are based on historic spending costs in the practice plus an amount reflecting Department of Health data on rises in prescribing costs and volume. Allowance is also made for practices with patients who receive particularly expensive medication. Some practices raised their prescribing costs when they knew indicative budgeting was to be introduced, to give themselves room for manoeuvre when the IPA was assigned. Thus, in the first year of IPAs, high cost practices got large IPAs and low-cost practices low ones. Practices which had increased their spending in anticipation were delighted. However, now that we are into the third year of the system, most FHSAs have levelled things out, and an FHSA or regional average amount has been assigned for each Astro PU. It is easier to increase prescribing than to reduce it, so some high-spending practices are now struggling somewhat.

Fundholders are given a true budget based on their historic spend, in the same way that IPAs are calculated for non-fundholding practices. For first wave fundholders, the budgets were more generous than they have been for succeeding waves. Many were able to make large savings in their drug budgets, which could help finance improvements to the premises or patient care. With each succeeding year, however, the possibility of making savings has been reduced by smaller budgets, and fourth wave fundholders will find it hard to save

Peristaltic Dysfunction in Gastro-oesophageal Reflux Disease

Peter J Kahrilas

Interest in oesophageal motor dysfunction in gastro-oesophageal reflux disease (GORD) has, until recently, focused on abnormalities of the lower oesophageal sphincter (LOS), in addition to LOS abnormalities, GORD may be associated with peristaltic dysfunction. In this article, the impact of peristaltic dysfunction on oesophageal volume clearance and acid clearance is discussed.

Assessment of normal peristalsis

Oesophageal peristalsis propels the contents of the oesophagus into the stomach. There are two ways of assessing peristaltic function which are commonly in use, barium oesophagrams and intraluminal manometry. Oesophagrams provide data on the timing and efficacy of bolus transport, while manometry yields data on the amplitude, duration and propagation velocity of peristaltic contractions.

Peristaltic abnormalities in patients with reflux disease

The amplitude of peristaltic contraction tends to be lower in patients with reflux disease compared with volunteer subjects or patient controls. More importantly perhaps, GORD patients also have an increased proportion of failed peristaltic contractions and in increased incidence of peristaltic contractions with hypotensive foci in the distal oesophagus. These abnormalities occur with increasing frequency as the severity of GORD increases, and both are associated with impaired oesophageal volume clearance. Failed peristaltic contractions result in low levels of volume clearance, while hypotensive peristaltic foci lead to impaired clearance as a result of retrograde escape. Retrograde escape occurs when the contractile amplitude is inadequate to achieve closure of the lumen behind the bolus: the peristaltic contraction may 'ride over' a segment of the oesophagus or a proportion of the bolus may escape in a retrograde direction through the area of contraction. The minimal peristaltic amplitude necessary to prevent retrograde escape varies depending on the region of oesophagus considered, but generally, contractions exceeding 30 mm Hg result in complete volume clearance of liquid barium. Peristaltic failure can either occur after the contraction successfully traverses the proximal oesophagus or there may be complete failure, such that a peristaltic contraction is not initiated after the swallow. Nonpropagated or simultaneous oesophageal contractions are associated with impaired oesophageal volume clearance. Analysing the peristaltic function of GORD patients with respect to those observations showed increased frequency of both failed peristaltic contractions and distal hypotensive foci paralleling the severity of the reflux disease.

Volume clearance vs acid clearance

The normal process by which the oesophagus is cleared of acid occurs as a two step process.

● Peristaltic contraction empties the oesophagus of acid or refluxate but does not result in restoration of the oesophageal mucosal pH to a neutral value, presumably because of hydrogen ions trapped in the fluid layer adherent to the oesophageal mucosa.

● Neutralisation of residual acid is accomplished in a stepwise fashion by swallowing saliva that contains a low concentration of bicarbonate.

If saliva is aspirated from the mouth and replaced with aliquots of water, the process of acid clearance is markedly prolonged, indicating that the mucosa is neutralised by saliva, not merely rinsed. Thus, for oesophageal acid clearance to proceed normally, effective volume clearance is necessary to remove all but a trace of the acidic refluxate and normal salivary function is necessary to neutralise the residue.

Significance of peristaltic dysfunction for oesophageal acid exposure

The development of peptic oesophagitis may ultimately depend on oesophageal acid exposure time, which is in turn the product of the reflux rate and acid clearance time. Acid clearance times in patients with GORD are, on the average, 2-3 times longer than those of normal individuals. As the process of acid clearance depends on both effective peristaltic function and normal salivation, impairments of either of these functions might be expected to prolong the process of acid clearance, with a resultant prolongation of oesophageal acid exposure time. Assuming a normal saliva production rate, the capacity of saliva to neutralise acid is in the order of 10-30 μEq/minute Gastric acid has about 100 μEq/ml of hydrogen ion, so salivary neutralisation alone would only account for relatively small volumes of refluxate. Similarly, it becomes apparent how minor aberrations in the completeness of volume clearance could account for the observed differences in the acid clearance times of some GORD patients as compared with control subjects.

This paper is one of series of articles on Motility, sponsored by Janssen Pharmaceutical Ltd. Others in the series available from Mr D.A. Cohen on 0235 777333.

much on this account. On top of the budget, regions have special contingency funds to cover some of the costs of patients who receive very expensive medicines.

Prescribing habits

The nature of prescribing is closely related to the individual doctor and his or her personality as well as the degree of illness in the practice population. Some doctors simply prescribe more, and more expensively, than others. Older doctors tend to be more conservative whereas younger ones may prefer to prescribe newer and more expensive drugs, many of which they have recently used in hospital training.

Practice manager's role

How can a practice manager improve practice prescribing and help to save costs? Between individual GPs, these can range from £11.50 to £28 per Astro PU. In a large practice, such differences tend to even out but in a smaller practice they may not. It is therefore important to encourage the doctors to look at their prescribing habits and be aware of the drug costs they are incurring.

The practice formulary

A practice formulary is invaluable. The partners should examine particular groups of drugs and decide which they are prepared to use. This involves discussion of effectiveness, side-effects, familiarity with the drugs, and costs. A good way to start is to study the PACT Level 3 report. This will show the drugs most often prescribed and, therefore, those which should be in the formulary. These should be listed according to their use with all the partners agreeing to the list, which should make some allowance for individual preferences.

As new drugs or drugs prescribed by hospital consultants which are not listed may have to be prescribed, the formulary should be regularly reviewed. It is a guide, not a tablet of stone.

Pharmaceutical and medical advisers

All FHSAs have independent medical advisers (many of them GPs) and most have pharmaceutical advisers (usually pharmacists), appointed and funded by the Department of Health to help control drug expenditure. They will visit practices about once a year to discuss prescribing, and can be very helpful. Their remit is to help to make prescribing effective and economical and they have up-to-date information on each practice's prescribing. They will be happy to supply the practice with graphs of trends in all aspects of prescribing over the previous two or three years, and will visit the practice, if asked, to discuss prescribing. Their aim is to educate, not to police. The practice manager should encourage the partners to seek such visits and should remind the advisers about patients on exceptionally expensive treatments.

Generic prescribing

A practice should prescribe generically as far as possible because generics are usually cheaper than the chemically identical brand name products. The generic (non-proprietary) names appear in the BNF or MIMS. If a generic is prescribed, the pharmacist may dispense any brand of the drug, usually that available at the best price or one he has in stock, thus saving time as well as cost.

An FHSA for a medium-sized town has calculated that it could save £2 million of its prescribing bill if all practices prescribed generically. But before instituting a generic policy, practice members should read the BNF guidelines on prescribing.

Repeat prescribing

The practice manager should take charge of the repeat prescription system, with the help of one of the partners. Repeat prescribing accounts for two thirds of prescribing costs. A well-managed system will enable repeat prescriptions to be both more rational and effective, and will save money. Whenever possible, repeat prescriptions should be attributed to and monitored by the doctor who instituted the repeat. A good system ensures that patients receive the correct drugs in the right doses and highlights patients who are taking more or less medicine than the doctor has prescribed. This helps to avoid side-effects from under- or over-dosing, minimises wastage and ensures that patients receive the best treatment. More drugs are wasted through inefficient repeat prescribing than in any other way.

Conclusion

A practice manager can do much to back up the prescribing skill of the doctors, to the benefit of the patients in improved health and to the practice in reduced costs. In fundholding practices, savings made in prescribing may be used to buy other services.

Nursing and Residential Homes

Pauline Ford

Continuing care for older people is increasingly provided in the community and those who need it will often receive nursing and/or residential care within a private or voluntary sector establishment.

This change has taken place against a changing population structure, a climate of rationing and funding restraint and a political philosophy which emphasises personal responsibility for health.[1]

Older people are the major consumers of NHS care, with 48 per cent of all NHS spending on this age group. The very elderly (those aged over 85) represent 1 per cent of the population but consume 8 per cent of NHS resources.[2] It is clear that older people will increasingly rely on the private and voluntary sector to meet their care needs. Demographic changes have been viewed with concern by health and social policy analysts and politicians, not least because of the financial consequences.

The current debate on health versus social care issues leads to consideration of nursing needs, what they are and how they should be provided. Much of the argument is finance-driven and many nurses have voiced concern that the older person's need of nursing is coming second to cost implications. This chapter therefore focuses on both nursing and residential homes; it covers the legal requirements and definitions and offers information on nursing, because general practitioners and practice managers may well be involved in these issues.

From April 1993, local authorities will fund community care and care managers (local authority employees) will assess the needs of older people and allocate resources.[3] Ideally, care managers will involve the older person, family carers and professional carers in that assessment.

Many social services departments have drawn up criteria for

admission to nursing homes which demonstrate that people resident in homes will have a much higher dependency than previously and are therefore likely to need skilled nursing and increased medical care. Indeed, it has been anticipated that direct admission to nursing homes from accident and emergency departments could occur when an older person is assessed as not requiring acute medical care.

If a resident needs continuous skilled nursing, physiotherapy or chiropody, there will be further costs. These services are currently free for people receiving care in hospitals, NHS nursing homes and in their own homes. Dependency is especially significant for those older people who have mental health needs. Many members of the Royal College of Nursing report that they have received limited training and education in identifying and meeting the mental health needs of this client group; generally, trained nurses working in the private sector feel particularly vulnerable. The College has therefore published guidelines for nurses on assessing older people.[4] Staffing levels in nursing and residential homes are prescribed by the registering authority, the health authority in the case of nursing homes and the local authority for residential homes. Each health and local authority has the power and responsibility to register and inspect all premises registered under the Registered Homes Act, 1984.[5]

Part 1 of this Act refers to residential homes and Part 2 to nursing homes. The homes registered under Part 1 are known as 'residential homes' and are registered and inspected by the local authority. They do not include nursing homes, which are registered under Part 2 and are registered and inspected by the district health authority.

Some homes are registered under both Parts 1 and 2, by both the health and the local authorities. An authority will usually appoint an inspector, who may also take on the role of registration officer and is thus involved in all the work associated with establishing a home before its registration. Charges are made for these services.

A registration officer can be involved from the start in either a flat site or an old mansion visit, before any plans are drawn up, through to the final stages of opening the home. This involves many meetings, discussions and site visits with the registration officer and representatives of statutory agencies such as the local building control, fire authority, health and safety executive and environmental health officers.

Both the owner of the home and the person in charge of the home must be 'fit' persons. It is for the registration officer to take up references and to determine that the business plan is realistic and viable.

The expertise, facilities and services of the David Lewis Centre for epilepsy at Warford, Cheshire, are of ever-increasing importance to General Practitioners, paediatricians and other consultants.

Founded in 1904 as a 'village' community, it is Britain's leader in the residential assessment, care and treatment of men, women and children suffering from epilepsy and associated disorders.

The objective, as far as is humanly possible, is to achieve stabilisation and return to the community.

At a recent conference held at the Centre, GPs were told that an average General Practice with 2,000 patients could expect up to 20 patients to have epilepsy – and that National Health Service assistance was surprisingly small, as it was regarded as a non-clinical condition.

Yet there are around 350,000 people in the UK with epilepsy. It is the second most common neurological disorder after migraine, and is as prevalent as diabetes.

The Centre is a registered charity, relying on public appeals, donations and legacies for the continued improvement of quality of life for residents and to maintain its leading position. Only operating costs are met by referral fees from Health, Education and Social Services authorities.

None the less, the Centre is extending its facilities to help those responsible for the treatment of people with epilepsy.

The EEG Department's services are available to GPs etc, at reasonable cost, for diagnosis and assessment, assisting treatment. The facilities include routine EEG, Brain Mapping, Ambulatory Monitoring, Video Telemetry, Evoked Potential, and Sphenoidal EEG.

In conjunction with the University of Manchester and Manchester Royal Infirmary, the Centre has established a model Epilepsy Clinic catering for out-patients drawn from a wide geographical area.

For details and brochure contact: Hugh Thompson, Chief Executive, The David Lewis Centre, Mill Lane, Warford, Near Alderley Edge, Cheshire SK9 7UD. Phone: Mobberley (0565) 872613. Fax: (0565) 872829.

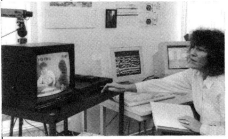
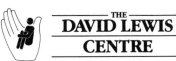

Implementation of the recommended staffing levels is one of the conditions of registration, which form a key part of registration and breach of which could lead to legal action. Other conditions apply to the number of residents and the category of the service to be provided. All such information is embodied in the condition of registration and no changes can be made without the agreement of the registering authority, although the home owner can appeal.

Monitoring of the home is a key part of the inspector's role. Statute states that all nursing homes must be inspected at least twice yearly, although many homes receive more visits than this. In legal terms, the inspector is responsible, acting as an officer of the registering authority and therefore the Secretary of State, for ensuring that there is no breach of the legislation or the conditions of the registration. In practice, inspectors find themselves doing much more than this, depending on the resources available.

As part of inspection monitoring is to establish that residents need nursing care, it is often the nurse inspector who is responsible for defining nursing care and deciding whether a resident requires it on either a continuous or intermittent basis. Currently, most of those with continuous nursing needs are cared for in nursing homes and those with intermittent need in residential homes, with nursing provided by community nurses.

In a dual registered home, it is permissible for those with both nursing and residential care needs to take up residence. This has the added benefit of enabling all care needs to be met in the one home, without having to move from one to another as their care needs change. The Royal College of Nursing has highlighted dual registration as a way of providing care that can meet peoples' changing needs[7] and has called for the barriers to dual registration to be removed.

The emphasis in residential homes is on maintaining well-being and independence. There is no legal requirement to employ nurses. The United Kingdom Central Council (UKCC), the governing body of nursing, recognises that there are ambiguities in the employment of nurses in the personal social service in general and the residential care sector in particular.[8] While many residential home proprietors do employ nurses (and may be nurses themselves), their employees are employed as carers, not nurses. However, many nurses working in residential homes feel they rely on their nursing experience. The UKCC expects that employers will recognise the advantages to the personal social services and residential care sectors which result from the employment of registered nurses. Nursing homes must be under the charge of a registered nurse or a registered medical practitioner.

There should be sufficient staff to provide skilled nursing to all residents.

On the face of it, the distinction between these two forms of provision appears clear, but older people do not necessarily fall conveniently into either category and, in any case, have changing needs. This has become especially noticeable as the balance between hospital and community care has changed. Definitions of continuing care needs vary and most health authorities now provide fewer continuing care beds for the elderly.

Most older people will benefit at some time from skilled nursing. In the residential home setting, there is need for some working definition of nursing which differentiates between what is done in the course of ordinary caring and activities which require greater knowledge and skill.

Focusing on tasks alone is unhelpful. Many are undertaken by nurses and non-nurses in a simply humanitarian response to people in need. Many people learn to care for themselves or their dependents. Ideally, care in the residential setting should be given by someone best known to the client, having the best caring relationship with them and the best possible professional knowledge and expertise. But it is inappropriate to define nursing in relation to tasks and techniques. The chief difference between nursing care, care from a nursing assistant, and personal care is not what is done but who is doing it. The vital difference is that the nurse has been fully trained, has a registration that gives her a legal right to her title, and is accountable to the UKCC.

In the past, people went into residential care when they were much younger than they do now, and there may not have been the same need for nursing intervention. Today's residents, however, are often in their late 80s or their 90s before admission becomes necessary. They are usually much frailer, and when they have a health problem it can need urgent attention.

The residential care nurse has a preventive and health promotion role, enabling the residents to maintain as much dignity and independence as they can; preventing ill health, controlling pain, promoting quality of life, and anticipating need, in line with an overall care plan.

The nurse is trained to provide:

Support and maintenance – residents and their relatives often feel reassured by the presence of a registered nurse, who can explain the problems that arise with ageing and offer practical, manageable solutions.

General management – ensuring that there are enough staff of the right calibre and that there are enough of the necessary materials.

Safe storage, control and administration of medicines – the registered nurse offers expertise on the need for medication and its effects on the clients.

Pre-admission assessment and continuing assessment – this can be enhanced by the professional experience of the registered nurse.

Ensuring an adequate diet – individual preference and the right to choice and control must be respected.

The nurse can use professional skills and knowledge to assess each resident's health and well-being. This will often make hospital admission unnecessary. Residents are not acutely ill and do not usually need medical or hospital care, but they are likely to have health and nursing needs which can benefit from intermittent nursing intervention. Nurses are also qualified to deal with the dying and their relatives and support the staff at such times.

The nursing or residential home can act as a bridge between hospital and the community. They can support hospitals by providing rehabilitation in a caring and supportive environment and support the community by offering respite and continuing care. Nurse specialists in homes, perhaps attached to local hospital units, can do much to ensure that older people receive the care they need and do not become unnecessarily dependent.

New Health and Safety Regulations

Norman Ellis

The Health and Safety at Work (HSW) Act is essentially a piece of enabling legislation which allows detailed parliamentary regulations to be enacted, and then promulgated and enforced by the Health and Safety Executive (HSE). These regulations lie at the heart of most activity in the health and safety field, spelling out in detail what is expected of employers.

Chapter 5.3 outlined the key principles of the main legislation; this chapter describes six new sets of HSW regulations which came into force on 1 January 1993. They apply to almost all kinds of work, including general practice, setting out in great detail how employers should protect both their employees and others, including members of the public.

These new regulations both implement EC directives and update existing health and safety law. They cover:

- general health and safety management;
- work equipment safety;
- manual handling of loads;
- workplace conditions;
- personal protective equipment;
- display screen equipment.

Most of the duties laid down by these regulations are not completely new; they merely clarify what is already health and safety law and make it more explicit. Any practice which is already complying with the HSW Act should easily be able to cope with the new regulations. But there are some new approaches, especially regarding the manage-

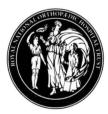

R N O H T

The Royal National Orthopaedic Hospital, was founded in 1905 with the amalgamation of London's three specialist orthopaedic Hospitals into a single centre of excellence and can thus trace its history back over 150 years, to 1838 when the Royal Orthopaedic Hospital was founded.

Teaching is inherent to the Hospital's work and the specialist training provided in all disciplines is in great demand both in this country and abroad. The RNOH, working closely with the University of London's Institute of Orthopaedics, forms the hub of the country's most comprehensive training programme for orthopaedic surgeons.

The institutional link with the Institute of Orthopaedics is of particular importance to the Hospital. Through the Institute's Biomedical Engineering Department the hospital, as part of the London Bone Tumor service, has pioneered limb preserving treatments through the use of massive and "growing" prostheses. Using CAD-CAM techniques bespoke implants and joint replacements are designed and manufactured which support the highly specialised programme for the revision of failed or worn joint replacements, including a growing demand for secondary revisions.

The Hospital has the largest Scoliosis Unit in Europe and in addition to surgical interventions, new conservative techniques have been developed which are particularly useful in infantile scoliosis. The purpose-built Spinal Injuries Unit and Rehabilitation Centre allows patients to be treated through the acute, rehabilitative and reintergrative phases of spinal injury. It includes the only purpose-built sports facility in Europe which actively integrates the disabled and the able bodied through sporting and other activities.

There are units specialising in most areas of orthopaedics including, Peripheral Nerve Injury, Shoulder Surgery, Joint Replacement, Paediatric Surgery, "Problem Backs" which have failed to respond to other treatment of the lumber spine as well as Hand, Foot and Knee surgery. In addition to the purely orthopaedic services there are services specialising in the treatment of Metabolic Bone Disorders, Rehabilitation, Rheumatology and a Tissue Viability Unit which specialises in the management of pressure sores.

The Hospital has two sites, a central London out-patient department which is easily accessible from all of the main line rail terminii, and both out- and in-patient facilities at Stanmore in north London. Because of the ease of access to the Bolsover Street site, 30 yards of Great Portland Street Underground, the Hospital can offer routine radiological investigations and physiotherapy services to GP Fundholders. Such services might be of interest to patients who work in central London as they would avoid taking time off from work to attend a local hospital.

ment of health and safety as such, and the use of VDUs, which practice managers may have to take into account.

General health and safety management

These new regulations set out broad general duties which, of course, apply to general practices. They aim to improve health and safety management and employers who are conscientious in their approach to health and safety should have no difficulty in getting to grips with them.

The regulations require employers to:

- assess the risk to the health and safety of their employees and anyone else who may be affected by their work, in order to identify any necessary preventive and protective measures. Employers with five or more employees should write their risk assessment down;

- make arrangements for putting into practice the preventive and protective measures that follow from this risk assessment: they should cover planning, organisation, control, monitoring and review (ie the management of health and safety). Again, any GP with five or more employees (do not forget that each part-time employee counts as one and also to include GP trainees or part-time clinical assistants) must put these arrangements in writing;

- carry out health surveillance of employees when appropriate;

- appoint a competent person (normally an employee) to help devise and apply the protective steps that the risk assessment shows to be necessary;

- set up emergency procedures;

- give employees information on health and safety matters;

- cooperate on health and safety matters with other employers sharing the same premises (eg the DHA or health board);

- make sure employees have adequate health and safety training and are capable enough at their job to avoid risk;

- give whatever health and safety information temporary staff need to meet their specific needs.

These regulations also:

- place duties on all employees to follow health and safety instructions and report danger;

- extend current health and safety law which requires employers to consult employees' safety representatives and provide facilities for them.

All these general duties exist alongside the more specific ones laid down in other health and safety regulations, including the new ones described below. Of course, this does not mean you have to do things twice. For example, if an employer has already made a risk assessment to comply with the Control of Substances Hazardous to Health (COSHH) Regulations, there is no need to repeat the exercise to comply with these new general management regulations.

Provision and use of work equipment

These regulations pull together and tidy up various laws governing equipment used at work; instead of piecemeal legislation covering particular kinds of equipment in different industries, these:

- place general duties on all employers;

- list minimum requirements for work equipment to deal with selected hazards which apply across all industries and sectors.

In general, these regulations make explicit what is already provided for elsewhere in current legislation or in good practice. If you have well chosen and well maintained equipment you should not need to do any more. Guidance on the regulations reinforces this point. Although some older equipment may need to be upgraded to meet the minimum requirements, you have until 1997 to do the necessary work. You should not allow yourself to be bamboozled by any local tradesmen who try to frighten you into employing them to undertake health and safety checks.

> 'Work equipment' is broadly defined to include everything from a hand tool, through machines of all kinds, to a complete plant such as an oil refinery. 'Use' includes starting, stopping, installing, dismantling, programming, setting, transporting, maintaining, servicing and cleaning.

The general duties of these regulations require general practices to:

- take into account the working conditions and hazards in the surgery when choosing equipment;

- make sure equipment is suitable for the use intended and that it is properly maintained;

- give adequate information, instruction and training.

Specific requirements cover:

- guarding dangerous parts of machinery (replacing current law on this);

- maintenance arrangements;

- dangers caused by equipment failure;

- parts and materials at high or very low temperatures;

- control systems and devices;

- isolation of equipment from power sources;

- physical stability of equipment;

- lighting;

- warnings and markings.

These regulations implement an EC directive on protecting workers. Other directives set out the conditions which much new equipment must satisfy before it can be sold in EC member states. These will be implemented in the UK by Trade and Industry Department regulations. Equipment which satisfies these other directives on standards should also meet many of the specific requirements listed above.

Manual handling operations

These regulations replace patchy, old-fashioned and largely ineffective legislation with a modern ergonomic approach to the problems of manual handling. They are important because the incorrect handling of loads causes many injuries, resulting in pain, time off work and even permanent disablement.

They apply to any manual handling operations which may cause injury at work; these should have been identified by the risk assessment carried out under the general health and safety management regulations described above. They include not only lifting loads, but also lowering, pushing, pulling, carrying or moving them, whether by hand or other bodily force. Again, these regulations are supported by general guidance.

There are health care areas where staff are at risk in this respect. An obvious example is nursing.

Employers have to take three key steps:

- avoid hazardous manual handling operations when reasonably practicable;

- assess adequately any hazardous operations that cannot be avoided;

- reduce the risk of injury as far as practicable.

Health, safety and welfare at the workplace

These regulations tidy up a lot of existing legislation, replacing some 35 pieces of old law, including parts of the Factories Act 1961 and the Offices, Shops and Railway Premises Act 1963. They are much easier to understand and make it far clearer what is expected.

These regulations cover many aspects of health, safety and welfare in the workplace, setting general requirements in four broad areas:

1 *Working environment*

- temperature;

- ventilation;

- lighting including emergency lighting;

- room dimensions;

- suitability of workstations.

2 *Safety*

- safe passage of pedestrians and vehicles (eg traffic routes must be wide enough and properly marked);

- windows and skylights (safe opening, closing and cleaning);

- transparent/translucent doors and partitions (use of safe material and marking);

- doors, gates and escalators (safety devices);

- floors (construction and maintenance, obstructions and slipping and tripping hazards);

- falls from height;

- falling objects (eg from cupboards or shelves).

3 *Facilities*

- toilets;

- washing, eating and changing facilities;

- clothing storage;

- seating;

- rest areas (and arrangements in them for non-smokers);

- rest facilities for pregnant women and nursing mothers.

4 *Housekeeping*

- maintenance of workplace, equipment and facilities;

- cleanliness;

- removal of waste materials.

You should ensure your premises comply with the regulations, but this does not have to be completed until 1996 for an existing surgery. Other people connected with the premises (eg the owner of a building which is leased to one or more employers or self-employed people) also have to ensure that requirements falling within their control are satisfied. Again, these regulations are supported by an approved code of practice.

Personal protective equipment

These regulations set out sound principles for selecting, providing, maintaining and using personal protective equipment (PPE).

Definition of 'personal protective equipment':

all equipment designed to be worn or held to protect against a risk to health or safety. It includes most types of protective clothing and equipment such as eye, foot and head protection, safety harnesses, life jackets and high visibility clothing. There are some exceptions, eg ordinary working clothes and uniforms (including clothes provided for food hygiene), those provided for road transport (eg crash helmets), and sports equipment.

PPE should be relied upon only as a last resort. But where risks are adequately controlled by other means, the employer has a duty to provide suitable equipment, free of charge, for all employees exposed to those risks. PPE is suitable only if it is appropriate for the risks and the working conditions, takes account of staff needs and fits them properly, gives adequate protection and is compatible with any other PPE they may wear.

Employers also have duties to:

- assess the risks and PPE they intend to issue to ensure that it is suitable;

- maintain, clean and replace PPE;

- provide storage for PPE when not being used;

- ensure PPE is properly used;

- give training, information and instruction on its use.

All new PPE must comply with an EC directive on design, certification and testing. This is implemented in the UK by regulations made by the Trade and Industry Department, but employers are allowed to use PPE bought before these regulations were implemented.

VDU health and safety

Unlike most of the regulations outlined above, the Health and Safety (Display Screen Equipment) Regulations do not replace old legislation, but cover a new area of work activity. Working with VDUs is not generally risky, but it can lead to muscular skeletal problems, eye fatigue and mental stress. Problems of this kind can be overcome by good ergonomic design of equipment, furniture, the working environment and the tasks performed.

The regulations apply to VDUs where there is a 'user', ie an employee who habitually uses it as a significant part of normal work. They cover equipment used for the display of text, numbers and graphics regardless of the display process used.

Employers' duties include:

- assessing VDU workstations and reducing risks which are identified;

- making sure workstations satisfy minimum requirements set for the VDU itself -- keyboard, desk and chair, working environment and task design, and software;

- planning VDU work so that there are breaks or changes in activity;

- providing information and training for VDU users.

VDU users are also entitled to appropriate eye and eyesight tests, and to special glasses if they are needed and normal ones cannot be used. Again, these regulations are supported by detailed guidelines.

Part Five

Managing Premises and Equipment

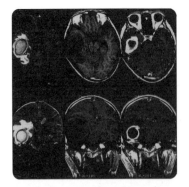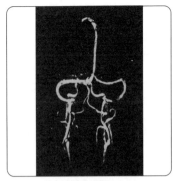
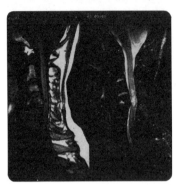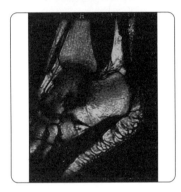

Now showing in London's West End.

Magnetic Resonance Imaging offers one of the clearest and most detailed aids to diagnosis and the monitoring of treatment.

The Queen Square Imaging Centre was opened in 1985 being the first direct referral MR Centre in the UK, providing a service for most clinical specialties which is available to everyone.

Queen Square has continued to invest in state-of-the-art MR scanning technology to enable it to offer the highest quality service to referring doctors and their patients.

We pride ourselves on providing a choice of convenient appointments with care and concern for our patients.

For referral, appointments or more information please telephone the centre on

071-833 2513.

Queen Square Imaging Centre

8-11 QUEEN SQUARE, LONDON WC1N 3AR. FAX: 071-837 8074.

Premises, Equipment and Maintenance

Angela Scott

Introduction

It is clear that the latest National Health Service reforms are driven by primary care and that practice management, still a young profession at around 20 years old, is under pressure to ensure the delivery of a more sophisticated, varied and value-for-money service at local level.

With this demand, and with management expertise developing at an unprecedented rate in general practice, so the requirement to operate from well planned, well organised and well equipped premises becomes more important than ever.

Premises

Managers in general practice have been most fortunate in that local, regional and national networking groups have been one of the strengths of the profession for many years. Experience has shown that contacts made in such forums can be very useful when a building project is planned. There seems little point in a practice 're-inventing the wheel' when building a surgery, so the job of the manager must be to gather useful information from other practices on any mistakes they may have made, and to seek advice on design, materials used, favoured architects and good building contractors.

A business plan contains the aims of a practice for an average of five years ahead, and its contents should be reviewed, and amended as appropriate, at least once a year. To meet the present and future needs

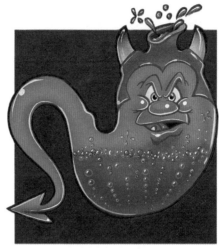

When excess stomach acid causes your patients grief,
choose a treatment that's effective, rapid-acting,
pleasant tasting, sugar-free and with a low sodium content.

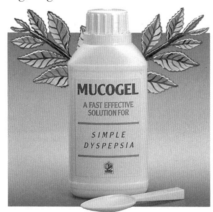

Thank goodness
MUCOGEL
Aluminium and Magnesium Hydroxides

A fast, effective solution for simple dyspepsia

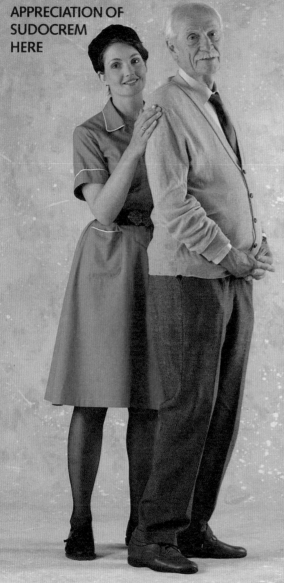

APPRECIATION OF SUDOCREM HERE

PREVENTS IRRITATION HERE

Sudocrem's been working for years, to soothe, heal and protect your incontinent patients against the associated misery of dermatitis.

Containing benzyl alcohol – an antiseptic and mild local anaesthetic[1], Sudocrem starts by rapidly soothing the skin. Its combination of zinc oxide, benzyl benzoate and benzyl cinnamate carry on to actively promote healing[2,3,4] while a natural and hypo-allergenic barrier helps prevent incontinence dermatitis recurring.

It's also useful for other forms of skin problems such as pressure sores, eczema and nappy rash.

Remember Sudocrem – a routine application can prevent a lot of irritation all round.

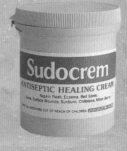

PHARMAX COMMUNITY CARE

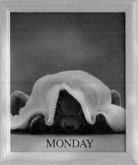

MONDAY

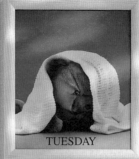

TUESDAY

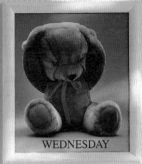

WEDNESDAY

INFACOL CAN HELP RESTORE

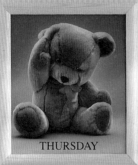

THURSDAY

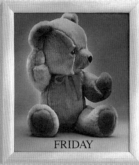

FRIDAY

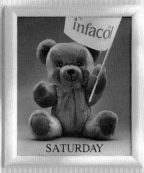

SATURDAY

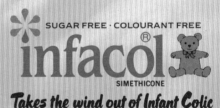

SUNDAY

THE PEACE

The piercing cries of a baby with colic can be distressing for the whole family. But by prescribing Infacol you can provide progressive relief for the symptoms right from birth.

Infacol contains Simethicone which encourages small bubbles of trapped gas to coalesce, aiding their expulsion.

In a double-blind placebo controlled study 0.5ml of Infacol given before feeds significantly reduced both the frequency and severity of attacks after several days of treatment.[1]

When Infant colic disturbs the peace, regular use of Infacol offers effective, progressive relief.

SUGAR FREE · COLOURANT FREE

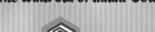

infacol ®

SIMETHICONE

Takes the wind out of Infant Colic

PHARMAX
COMMUNITY
CARE

of doctors, patients and staff, the commitments, plans and ideas in the report must be examined and closely met.

Vision and innovation

It is often not cost-effective or feasible to buy extra land when planning a building project. Consequently, the design of new premises, with the envisaged expansion of primary care services, must contain vision. New buildings must incorporate innovative features which allow for changes to be made to the interior layout as times change and valuable space needs to be gained or room use altered. Subject to planning restrictions, the shape and pitch of the roof design is important, to give the option in future of a loft conversion scheme with minimal disruption and expense. Or, perhaps, the new construction should be strengthened to allow the addition of further floors. The architect should be well briefed about your wishes and will advise accordingly. He or she can also help with decisions about the positioning of power and telephone points, with scale drawings for each area, along with cardboard cut-outs of desks, chairs and other large furniture, such as couches. These will help to focus on the available space and the best way to use it. It is advisable to discuss with the architects the design and installation of a ducting system to run through the premises, to include electrical, telephone and computer cabling, for maximum effectiveness and adaptability.

Internal design

The consulting room

These aspects, particularly as they affect the use of a computer terminal and printer, are important in the design of the consulting room. Internal walls must be soundproof and, to minimise interruptions during consultations, it is a good idea to introduce small hatch-type recesses in the walls, to allow for the passing of urgently needed medical records and messages -- and cups of coffee. Frosted glass windows give plenty of natural light and allow flexibility in fitting blinds or curtains. The combination of a cheerful decor with, perhaps, a separate examination room to soften the obvious clinical emphasis, allows other professionals to work in these rooms between surgery times.

Treatment space

It is clear that a good design and some improvisation are needed in the clinic and treatment areas of the surgery to take the developing role of the practice nurse into account. With more minor surgical procedures and small operations being performed at primary care level, there is a need for facilities for general practitioners and their nurses to work efficiently together. To meet this, it is necessary to include double sinks with elbow taps for a high standard of hygiene and, in the interests of health and safety, to build in a lockable eye-level fridge among an ample range of lockable cupboards and drawers. The setting in which patients are seen either individually or in group sessions is all-important. The allocation of open space, with soundproof room dividers, may meet this demand, while a treatment suite with some curtained cubicles, combined with a private room, may give greater flexibility. Clearly, closer monitoring of chronic diseases such as diabetes, asthma, coronary heart disease, thyroid malfunction, epilepsy and hypertension is developing fast in primary care, and a well-planned working environment will be needed for the practice nurse to play a full role in providing care.

Expanding primary care services

In building, refurbishing, extending and improving premises, the practice must look at plans for developing further in-house services and consider the needs of the visiting hospital consultant, chiropodist, counsellor, speech therapist, dietician and physiotherapist, and there is growing support for offering some forms of alternative medicine too. As we strive to provide seamless care for our patients, and to achieve closer links within the primary health care team, health visitors and district nurses attached to the practice should be offered a room in the surgery as a base from which to work. While some practices may decide to have a multi-purpose suite, others may find that, as space is limited, a room-use rota has to be maintained, with the allocation of any necessary storage space.

The dispensary

The practice may be fortunate enough to house a dispensary. This popular facility needs to be of easy access to patients, but care must be taken to ensure the safety and security of staff. Secure windows with toughened glass, solid doors, a lockable patient hatch, a floor safe for dangerous drugs and an alarm system with a panic button, should ensure that the dispensary and staff are protected from crime. If a practice expects its in-house pharmacy will be offering over-the-counter medicines to practice patients in future, ample storage space will be needed. Here, innovation and improvisation come into play, to allow for further shelving and cool storage facilities as demand increases for a wider range of products.

The reception area

General practice, like the rest of the National Health Service, has become much more competitive. According to marketing professionals, it costs six times more to attract a new customer than to keep an existing one, so we must look to our patients' needs in order to make an impact in the market place. We must exploit every opportunity and, faced with the challenge of improving the practice generally, should give priority to the design of the reception desk. A prime concern in a commercially viable general practice nowadays is in continuing to emphasise customer care; we must welcome the approaching end of an era in which patients may have to shout their personal details to the receptionist through a glass screen. In looking to provide a welcoming reception counter, many new or renovated surgeries favour an open plan design, like those often found in modern hotels. However, for matters of a confidential or perhaps embarrassing nature, patients need an area where they can speak to a member of staff privately; ideally, this should be a private room close to reception. Manual or computerised medical records must be maintained and filed, with an emphasis on easy access and retrieval. To have a good idea of the shape and size of the room, it is necessary to research methods for storing records securely, with due consideration to the system used.

The waiting area

To be most welcoming for patients, the waiting area should be brightly decorated, light, spacious, airy and comfortable, with a safe play area for children. Well placed power points for television, and perhaps video equipment, are useful, as is wall space for notices. It is worth noting that the cost of fixed seating for the waiting room is included in the total development costs, but such seating may limit flexibility in making good use of a large area.

Office space

The surgery's office areas need careful consideration as they need to house the practice manager, secretaries and clerical staff, including computer operators. Many new surgeries allow plenty of room for clinical work but give the management and clerical team too little space to work efficiently. There should be enough power and telephone points, strategically placed, in walls, floors and ceilings for present purposes and possible future needs. Experience suggests it may be best to follow the model of many large organisations which, rather than lose space with interior dividing walls, have chosen open-plan offices with portable acoustic screening to apportion space as tasks develop and teamwork grows. If the office area is upstairs, it may be useful to install a small elevator rather than have staff running up and down with medical notes.

The common room and library

In a 1990s practice, there should be a common room where practice staff can have coffee, meet, relax and have training sessions. There should also be space to make drinks and light refreshments, and for a staff cloakroom. A soundproof room-divider is invaluable here, allowing a quiet area in the common room to be closed off for private meetings or as a library or reference zone.

Special facilities

Disabled patients must not be forgotten when planning the width of doorways and the design and positioning of toilet facilities. It is clearly an advantage for all consulting space to be on the ground floor, but if this is not feasible, consider accommodating patients who cannot climb stairs in a ground floor room. A ramp may be needed at the entrance for wheelchairs, prams and pushchairs.

Housekeeping

Health and safety regulations and policy must be at the forefront of running a good professional healthcare service, with an emphasis on top standards of cleanliness and hygiene for patients and staff alike. It is essential to comply with legal requirements in providing lockable provision for clinical waste, including used needles, and for cleaning staff to store their materials and equipment safely and securely in a separate utility annexe off the kitchen.

Best use of current premises

Although many surgeries have improved in recent years, pressure on space is considerable and many health centres and surgeries have become cramped. The practice manager can use feasibility studies, under the cost rent or improvement grant schemes, to find the answer to this. In some places, consortia of several health care professionals, including dentists, pharmacists and general practitioners, have set up charity trusts to work with private developers in converting health centre premises into one-stop health complexes.

Many practices work in health centres owned by the district health authority or perhaps a community health care trust. These organisations have become more financially aware and may be interested in renting extra space that has perhaps been used for one particular activity or service, but not on a full-time basis.

There are also many practices which have secured, or are negotiating for, the purchase of the health centre where they are based. Many of these buildings are too small, run-down or inadequately equipped, but with guidance and support from the family health services authority or health board, a well-timed and managed project, combining the purchase of the site with planned alterations, can be financed as a complete package under the cost rent scheme.

Improvement grants

The improvement grant scheme may be used to help finance a modification or extension. It is designed to cover the addition of rooms, the conversion of a loft area, the improvement of toilet facilities, the extension of the telephone system, the installation of a security system or improvements in parking space. Again, the appropriate authority will give advice about funding, and the practice's business plan can be adjusted accordingly.

Equipment

The amount and type of equipment in a surgery will vary from practice to practice. But however well-planned and designed the premises are, appropriate funding for all necessary purchases is vital.

Some of the following items are termed fitments, and will, therefore, be included in the cost of a development or refurbishment.

Consulting rooms

Basic equipment

- workstation comprising desk, chair, VDU, screen stand, keyboard, quiet printer and foot stool if needed
- telephone (incorporating hands-free facility and patient calling mode)
- two patient chairs
- adjustable desk lamp
- blinds or curtains
- noticeboard and shelving
- wall-mounted height gauge (precisely placed)
- vanity hand basin
- towel hook
- stethoscope
- sphygmomanometer (including a selection of cuffs)
- auriscope
- peak flow meter with disposable tubes
- ophthalmoscope and otoscope
- hand-held dictating machine
- percussion hammer
- adult weighing scales
- panic button (connected to reception area)
- wall clock
- wastepaper bin
- used sharps bin
- tongue depressors and urine testing kit
- coat hook
- thermometers, oral and rectal

Specialised equipment

- spirometer
- nebuliser
- head mirror

Examination room

Basic equipment

- examination couch and blanket
- couch paper roll holder
- suspended curtain rail and couch curtain or free-standing screen
- step stool
- wall-mounted cold light source (luminaire)
- instrument trolley
- washbasin unit with hot and cold elbow mixer taps
- towel rail or hook and soap dispenser

- mirror
- eye chart (set up for correct distance in mirror)
- coat hook
- chair (for patients' belongings)
- clinical waste bin
- vaginal speculae and containers
- proctoscope (disposable or metal)

Specialist equipment

- foetal heart monitor (small doppler)
- cervical clamps

Treatment area

Basic equipment

- workstation comprising desk, chair, telephone, VDU, keyboard, screen
- stand, printer, and foot stool if needed
- two patient chairs
- an array of eye and low level lockable cupboards with drawers
- lengths of kitchen-style worktops

- steriliser/autoclave
- weighing scales
- wall-mounted height gauge
- height/weight conversion chart
- panic button (connected to reception area)
- eye chart
- stethoscope
- sphygmomanometer

- double sink and drainer fitted with hot and cold elbow mixer taps
- built-in lockable drugs, refrigerator and thermostat
- generous supply of double-sockets
- examination couch, blanket and pillow
- step stool
- couch paper roll holder
- a suspended rail and couch curtain or free standing couch screen
- coat hook
- mirror
- adjustable desk lamp
- wall mounted luminaire
- dressing and instrument trolleys

- clinical waste bin
- used sharps waste bin
- noticeboard and shelving
- ear syringe and tank and electric propulse ear syringe kit
- ophthalmoscope
- peak flow meter, charts and disposable tubes
- masks and gowns
- disposable gloves and aprons
- spatulae
- nasal speculum
- vaginal speculae and containers
- laryngoscope
- fire extinguisher

A basic instrument kit may include:

- scissors (all sizes)
- Spencer Wells forceps (all sizes)
- dissecting forceps
- splinter forceps
- crocodile forceps
- scalpal blade holder and blades
- suture removing instruments

- aural and nasal forceps
- currettes
- a range of other forceps (as needed)
- a range of sizes of kidney dishes
- mouth gag (for emergency)
- tongue forceps and tray
- a range of sizes of galley pots

Specialised equipment for use by either doctors or nurses

- electrocardiogram (ECG)
- haemoglobinometer
- microscope
- ambulatory BP machine
- TENS unit
- spirometer
- audiometer
- portable x-ray light box

- glucometer
- ESR tubes
- cauterising equipment
- smokerlyzer
- electric nebuliser
- cryoprobe
- portable ultra-sound scanner

Resuscitation kit

- portable oxygen cylinder
- a range of airways and masks
- resuscitation bag
- intravenous infusion set
- laryngoscope

- emergency aspirator
- endotracheal tubes
- intubation equipment
- emergency drugs (practice specified)

The above resuscitation kit may be purchased in a specially constructed suitcase or kept in a portable container to allow easy access for emergency situations both in and outside the surgery.

Reception desk

- built-in desking
- VDUs and keyboards
- telephones
- appointment books for surgeries and clinics

- below desk shelving for forms
- noticeboard
- chairs
- house plants

Records office

- shelf units or cabinets for filing MREs
- telephones
- VDUs and keyboards
- noticeboards and shelves
- town map
- white or blackboard and markers
- alarm unit for internal/ external security system
- message and visit book
- telephone directories
- safety step stool
- filing trays and boxes
- meter cupboards
- fuse box

Waiting area

- chairs or fixed seating
- noticeboards
- safe play area for children with toys, books, table and chairs
- TV (and perhaps video) with aerial point
- public address system
- coffee tables with magazines
- clear directional signs for toilets and consulting/ treatment room
- childproof power sockets
- fire extinguisher

Dispensary

- workstation comprising desk, chair, VDU, keyboard, medicine label and prescription printers, VDU stand and footstool if needed
- high and low level lockable cupboards and drawers
- kitchen-type work surfaces
- double sink and drainer
- built-in eye level drugs refrigerator and refrigerator
- floor-fitted safe for dangerous drugs
- modem for wholesale drug ordering
- tablet counter
- cash till
- measuring jars
- storage area for bottles, spoons and packaging
- secure cupboard for prescription pads and storage area for FP10 comps

---

Common room and library

- comfortable chairs
- white or blackboard with markers
- noticeboard
- shelving for books
- magazine rack
- storage for back numbers of medical journals
- coffee and/or dining table
- house plants
- coat hooks
- soundproof room divider
- wastepaper bin
- doctors' pigeon holes
- television and aerial point
- overhead projector
- flip chart and stand

Kitchen

- eye and low level cupboards and drawers
- double sink with hot and cold mixer taps and drainer
- wall-mounted microwave oven
- toaster
- kettle
- crockery and cutlery
- trays
- refrigerator
- filter coffee maker and teapot

Staff cloakroom and toilets

- secure locker-type cabinets
- coat hooks
- mirror
- male and female WC

Office space

We shall deal with the equipping of the office area, on the basis that each member of this group, regardless of status, requires their own basic equipment and also has a need to share the use of 'general items'.

General items

- computer central processing unit or, if the practice is using a networked computer system, a file server

- tape streamer with magnetic tapes

- facsimile machine

- guillotine

- electronic typewriter

- filing cabinets

- house plants, especially spider plants for putting moisture back into the atmosphere

- shredder

- laser printer

- telephone directories

- photocopier

- ionisers

- continuous power unit

- shelf units

- fire extinguisher

Each workstation comprises

- desk

- chair

- VDU

- copy holder

- keyboard

- VDU stand

- stapler

- hole punch

- stationery items

- calculator

- filing trays

NB Wrist supports, screen filters, footstools, desk lamps and anti-static mats should be supplied, if required, after health and safety assessment.

Multi-purpose rooms

It may be that the consulting or treatment rooms are also used for housing other in-house services such as physiotherapy, hospital consultant outreach clinics or a counsellor.

Here is some of the equipment that may be required by a

physiotherapist, though some items may be supplied under the agreed contract. Purchasing power will vary from practice to practice; many first-wave fundholders have spent savings on equipping the surgery with useful items, required to run an expanding range of services, for their patients.

Physiotherapy service

- ultrasound machine
- interferential machine
- TENS unit
- compact multi-gym

- hi-lo plinth
- portable traction unit
- foradic machine
- pulsed short-wave machine

General features which can benefit all users of the surgery premises include:

- a porch area or air-lock at all outside access doors;
- central heating system to allow individual thermostat use;
- a frost stat and seven-day clock for the heating system;
- British standards must be observed when fitting a fire alarm system;
- fluorescent lighting with diffusers;
- burglar alarm system connected to an outside source;
- power supply needs spike testing and voltage regulation;
- heavy-duty lockable door handles;
- a digital entry system on the rear door of the surgery;
- maintenance costs may be kept down by leaving walls of corridors and public areas with a brick facia.

Maintenance

A maintenance programme for both equipment and premises is necessary for a smoothly running organisation. Managers should also be aware of the legal and moral implications of accidents involving employees that may occur as a result of poorly maintained equipment.

Buildings

For a successful maintenance programme:

- implement a cleaning protocol, and include daily, weekly and quarterly tasks as well as 'spring cleaning';
- stress to staff the need to keep computer environments dust-free;
- have a planned programme of redecoration of both the interior and exterior of the premises;
- note dates that each room and area were decorated;
- organise a cleaning contract for regular treatment of carpets;
- if carpet is the floor covering in public areas, contract with an exchange laundry mat service to deliver a regular supply of clean porch floor and front-of-reception desk rugs;
- employ a part-time handyperson to change light bulbs regularly, do the gardening and keep the surgery well maintained;
- adhere strictly to fire regulations, paying particular attention to the blocking of doorways, exits and corridors.

Equipment

- keep handbooks for all equipment;
- hold annual servicing agreements on the burglar alarm, boiler and fire extinguishers;
- contract for daily help-line computer support, which includes comprehensive software and hardware computer maintenance;
- train staff in all aspects of health and safety regulations;
- implement a comprehensive health and safety policy;
- regularly check all electrical equipment, with particular attention to plugs and wiring;
- position equipment safely, without trailing wires;
- have a maintenance agreement for typewriters, shredders and photocopiers;
- organise a regular fire drill and fire alarm test;

- organise staff training in the safe use of all items of equipment.

A policy of good housekeeping at all levels will benefit the practice. The investment of time and money will make for a safer and happier environment.

Choosing a Laboratory

David Browning

The cultural change sweeping through the NHS is giving many general practices a new freedom to choose which services, including those from pathology laboratories, they will use. The ways in which laboratories perceive and give a service are changing accordingly. Any loss of work to a competing laboratory can mean less revenue so pathology laboratories, whether in the independent or the public sector, are seeking to attract work, while those in the NHS in particular are having to acquire new skills. They are having to learn to cultivate and retain custom and provide a service the customer requires. NHS pathology is no longer just provider led, but is becoming customer led, as has been the practice in the private sector for years. General practices are therefore likely to have the opportunity to choose the laboratory from which they buy a pathology service. They will probably receive a mass of information from several laboratory organisations and will have to choose between the laboratory it has been using and potential new suppliers which it will have to appraise.

We all constantly make purchasing decisions, based on such factors as convenience and quality and, of course, are unlikely to return to a provider after a bad experience with them. The same is now true with laboratories, and managers will have the opportunity to question the level of service to be provided and to ensure they get value for money. A manager will wish to assess the organisation as objectively as possible, but there will be subjective criteria too.

Total quality

Before inviting any organisation to tender for your pathology work it is essential to be clear what level of service you need. It should be

BIOLAB MEDICAL UNIT

Nutritional Clinical Biochemistry Laboratory

Central London (established 1984)

Biolab is a specialised clinical biochemistry laboratory providing a comprehensive range of nutritional analyses for medically qualified practitioners. The laboratory is run by qualified staff and subscribes to relevant quality control schemes.

In addition to the following tests, a number of other specialised profiles are also available (details available on request):

Vitamins	**Trace Elements**	**Toxic Metals**
Essential Fatty Acids	**Amino Acids**	**Gut Permeability**
Absorption Tests	**Gut Fermentation**	**Pesticides**

Experienced nursing staff provide a free phlebotomy service for patients attending the laboratory; alternatively many of the analyses can be performed on postal samples.

Please call the laboratory for a comprehensive list of the tests available, fees and sample requirements, or to discuss your specific needs.

Telephone: 071-636 5905/5959   Fax: 071-580 3910

Biolab Medical Unit provides a referral clinical laboratory service specialising in nutritional assessment of patients using a wide range of methods.

Research worldwide has shown that the assumption that "if you eat a balanced diet you can't be deficient in any micronutrients" is incorrect.

Since there are great variations in individuals' abilities to absorb dietary vitamins, minerals and essential fatty acids, some people can be deficient in one or more essential nutrients despite being on what would generally be considered an adequate diet. Furthermore, disease processes, medications, environmental and life-style factors also affect nutrient requirements.

It is now known that antioxidant vitamins and minerals and essential fatty acids play an important role in protecting against a range of diseases, including heart attack, stroke and certain types of cancer. Deficiencies can affect immune function, mental function, energy level, the menstrual cycle, ovulation, sperm production and so forth.

Use of the nutritional laboratory can give the clinician valuable guidance in advising patients on dietary requirements and nutritional supplementation programmes.

Regular workshops and seminars are held to help doctors learn how to make best use of the nutritional laboratory.

Since it was established in 1984, Biolab has performed nutritional tests for more than 60,000 patients, providing a wealth of research data. The doctors and biochemists at the unit regularly present their findings at international meetings and publish papers in peer review journals.

Biolab also provides at no charge, full test protocols to NHS hospital laboratories wishing to perform particular nutritional biochemical tests themselves.

possible to assess a laboratory's quantity and range of tests, and you will take account of the likely expansion, contraction or changes in its range of work. What problems have there been previously, such as delays in getting results or not getting them at all? Such issues need to be carefully recorded. Objectivity in recording is vital because it is easy to remember the occasional error but to forget the majority of occasions when the service was satisfactory. The potential supplier of a service may well have ideas on how it might be improved; this could include such options as providing the service in your surgery or clinic while using conventional laboratory staff. Other options will need to be discussed in the light of your requirements and budget.

There are three phases in the supply of the service – pre-analytical, analytical and post-analytical. Each is, of course, related to the others but is best described separately to help assessment. A purchasing manager or doctor should assess the factors, prioritise them, and use this as the basis for its questions to the potential supplier.

Pre-analytical

Laboratories rightly point out that the quality of any result depends on the quality of the specimens they receive. The importance the laboratory gives to this is a good guide to the quality of its total operation. It should have a booklet or brochure which contains guidance on how to collect specimens, what type of containers to use, how the laboratory is organised and on the scope of its work. Its service should be simple to use, with only a single request document for all your laboratory work, for instance, although histopathology and cytology will be exceptions to this rule. The laboratory should also give the names, positions and roles of senior staff and indicate from whom you can get advice on such matters as the supply of containers or dealing with complaints as well as discussing aspects of the service or interpretation of results. Such information should be readily available when required and will include up-to-date details of the turnaround time of test results, batching of less frequently requested tests and the availability of phlebotomy services at the laboratory site or in your clinic or surgery. How frequently are specimens collected and is this part of the service? What happens when you need urgent investigations? The information supplied must assure you of a quality service without constant recourse to telephone inquiries.

Analytical

This might seem difficult for a non-laboratory worker to assess, but all laboratories should have quality control data available for inspection and discussion. In addition, the quality of many analyses can be assessed by the use of External Quality Assessment. This is an independent system run by an outside agency which supplies samples of unknown concentration or content. The samples are analysed in the laboratory as if they were patient specimens and the results returned to the organiser who will write a report based on the results on the same material from a large number of laboratories. Over time, these will reveal a pattern of comparative performance. Is the one you propose to use a good, moderate or poor performer? Beware of the laboratory that always seems perfect – even the best organisation makes mistakes and admitting to and learning from them is a sign of strength, not weakness. The laboratory's senior staff should be willing to explain these analytical quality issues to you. The way the results on your patient are compared with the reference ranges quoted will be important.

Post-analytical

This phase is likely to be the most openly used to judge a laboratory's performance. In essence, it is the end result or product. Are the reports intelligible? Do they arrive on time? Is there a modem link between your computer and the laboratory? Can you interrogate it? What interpretation is available and how often and from whom? Can you get follow-up advice and discuss any problems with the appropriate senior staff? What is the response when a clinically significant or unexpected result occurs? These are the sort of questions to consider.

Licensing and accreditation

Although there are various licensing systems, including NAMAS, GLP Compliance and BS 5750, the most relevant to pathology laboratories is provided by Clinical Pathology Accreditation (UK) Ltd – CPA, which is managed by an independent non-profit making company whose directors come from all the main professional pathology bodies in the UK. Compliance with its standards and accreditation can be obtained after it has been visited by trained inspectors from the professions involved. Unconditional accreditation usually entails a detailed full day's inspection by two inspectors per pathology discipline. There are currently 44 standards in six sections with which an applicant laboratory must comply. These standards ensure that there are appropriately trained staff, that there is good analytical quality and that the service, as judged by other users, is satisfactory. Accreditation assures you that all the elements are in place to ensure a quality service at all stages. You may also be able to consult another user as a final check.

Added value

While analytical and non-analytical quality are essential, there are other aspects of the service which may help you distinguish between different laboratories. Do they regularly top-up supplies of replace-ment specimen containers? Will those responsible for the laboratory visit you regularly to monitor the progress of the contract, deal with any problems and adapt to your changing demands. How will they deal with an unusual occurrence or request? Do they provide a service outside normal working hours? Will the staff welcome a visit from you and show you around so that you and your staff can put faces to names and voices? What opportunities will be given for formal review? Such qualities may be the 'icing on the cake' to help you choose between one laboratory and another.

Finance

Quality costs money. If you have carefully specified the services you consider important, the laboratory should be able to provide a price list with a clear specification of what it proposes for you. If there are big differences in prices between one laboratory and another, there will be good reasons and you should find out what they are and in precisely what way the proposals vary. There might be substantial quality differences and you will need to look into these. Judicious questioning should enable you to come to a positive decision with confidence.

Choosing a laboratory should be the same as choosing any other expensive service or product. You must be clear about what you need

Table 5.2.1 *Choosing a laboratory*

Pre-analytical	Analytical
Description of service (handbook)	Quality control
Contact names	External Quality Assessment
Types of containers	Reference Ranges
Regular top-up	
Single request form	
Turnaround times	
Fax/Modem links	
Specimen transport	

Post-analytical

Report format
Interpretation/advice/follow-up
Accreditation
Monitoring/contract contact
Flexibility
Emergency services
Costs

and read the various proposals with care. The cheapest may not be the best or may not suit your requirements. It will be in your own interest to make a list of the issues you consider important. You may find it helpful to prepare a table like the one on the previous page (see Table 5.2.1).

Health and Safety in the Surgery

Norman Ellis

The duties arising from the Health and Safety at Work Act and its regulations are not difficult to apply and most surgery premises should meet their requirements. The legislation requires an employer (including a self-employed person) to provide and maintain a safe working environment and it establishes powers and penalties to enforce this.

Because surgeries are in the 'health services' grouping, they are inspected by a Health and Safety Executive (HSE) official not, as often assumed, by a local government environmental officer. The frequency of HSE inspectors' visits to surgeries is increasing. This chapter provides guidance on matters which an inspector may wish to discuss; it is not a definitive statement or interpretation of the law.

Employers' duties to staff

The Act's main aim is to make employers and employees conscious of the need for safety in all aspects of their day-to-day work. The most important duty, which every employer must fulfil, is:

'to ensure, so far as is reasonably practicable, the health, safety and welfare at work of all his employees'. (Health and Safety at Work Act 1974.)

The meaning of 'reasonably practicable' may be inferred from case law and the advice of HSE inspectors.

Any proceedings taken under the Act are criminal and any employee can report a breach of an employer's statutory duty to the HSE.

A Court's assessment of whether it is 'reasonably practicable' to avoid a particular hazard or risk of injury takes account of the cost of preventive action (particularly if an employer has few staff and limited resources) and weighs this against the risk of injury and its possible severity.

Written statement of safety policy

An employer should provide information, training and supervision for staff on health and safety matters. Unless there are fewer than five staff, the employer must provide a statement of general policy on health and safety and ensure it is implemented; employees should be consulted on its form and content. The HSE discourages the use of 'model' statements; employers should prepare their own and should not take the easy option of adopting a 'model' statement because that could discourage serious consideration of health and safety policy and its implementation.

However, contrary to this advice, here is a specimen written statement.

Health and safety in the practice

The partners' policy on health and safety in the surgery is to ensure that everyone's working environment is as safe and healthy as possible. As a member of the staff you are expected to support this aim.

Your employer is ultimately responsible for your health and safety, but you also have a legal duty to take reasonable care to avoid any action or working pattern which might cause injury to yourself, your colleagues or others using the surgery premises. In particular, you should not meddle with or misuse any clothing or equipment provided to ensure health and safety.

There are certain hazards you should know about:

- prams and cycles parked on the premises;
- medical equipment and instruments used in the consulting rooms;
- cooking utensils and equipment used in the staff restroom.

You must report any accident to the doctor in charge as soon as possible. You should write down what has happened and explain how the accident occurred, so that we can take steps to stop it happening again.

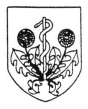
HERBAL MEDICINE

Herbal medicine is probably the oldest form of medicine known; it is also the most natural form of all existing disciplines today. There was, in essence, no difference originally between the food we consumed and the medicines we swallowed. Most vegetables and food plants we know nowadays are glorified editions, produced by the nursery grower, of the wild weeds our forefathers ate.

Modern herbal medicine, phytotherapy as it is called and now rapidly becoming known, is probably the only form of medicine most akin to orthodox medicine. It does not administer its treatment of the patient on the couch in the form of needles, joint manipulation, long or short wave therapy, but offers the treatment in a bottle of medicine. The great advantage of herbal medicine is that most people are able to "self medicate". Everyone can buy herbs, dried, in tablet form, as tincture etc. and experiment on themselves without any interference from a practitioner, and 61% of the British population has done so at least once in their lives, according to a public opinion poll of approximately three years ago.

The School of Phytotherapy (Herbal Medicine) at Bucksteep Manor, Bodle Street Green, Hailsham, East Sussex BN27 4RJ, now has a four year correspondence course for those wishing to set up in practice and a four year full-time course, also for those wishing to qualify as practitioners. People qualifying from these four year courses are able to deal in a very professional and competent way with most problems.

A visit to a phytotherapist (medical herbalist) may not be, in some instances, very much different to a visit to your orthodox practitioner. You will have a case-taking and probably a clinical examination.

The written statement may be included in each employee's employment contract. In a practice with fewer than five staff, the statement can be posted in a public place; it is not necessary to give everyone a copy.

Safety representatives

Safety representatives are usually appointed if an employer recognises a trade union; in general practice they are most likely to be in health centres where health authority staff work with practice staff. Safety representatives have considerable powers on health and safety matters: inspecting the workplace, enquiring into accidents, raising complaints directly with the employer and insisting on a joint staff-management safety committee being formed. They have a right to challenge the employer on all health and safety matters.

It has been proposed that safety representatives should be appointed where the staff are not unionised. Because the employer and staff share a duty to ensure health and safety, the Health and Safety Commission has suggested that staff should be involved in developing and promoting health and safety policy and procedures. Appointing safety representatives may not be practicable in a small practice. It may be sufficient for an employee (possibly the practice manager) to be appointed as the 'safety officer' to monitor health and safety.

Duties to others using the surgery

An employer must ensure the safety of anyone using the surgery, including patients, pharmaceutical representatives, visitors, builders, tradesmen and health authority staff. If the premises are owned by a private landlord or local health authority, the licence or lease may impose this duty upon the other party, who may also be liable if there is an accident.

The Act requires the practice to be run so as to ensure that all users of the premises are safe from risks of personal injury. For example, it is necessary to consider whether there are any potential hazards to elderly or infirm patients. The Occupier's Liability Act 1957 already lays down a 'common duty of care' owed to all persons using the premises.

Notifying accidents and dangerous occurrences

An employer should keep a record of accidents and, if he or she is the 'controller of the premises', notify the HSE of certain serious accidents to anyone using the premises.

Normally the employer, or the controller of the premises, will be responsible for reporting any accident. Although there may be circumstances where the owner of the premises and not the GP is held responsible, it is best to assume that the practice should notify the HSE.

Employees' responsibilities

Staff must take reasonable care of their own health and safety on the premises, and of the safety of other users of the premises who may be affected by their actions or omissions. They are expected to cooperate with the employer in carrying out these duties. Although the duties of employees technically apply 'while at work', it would be wise to assume that these also apply throughout the time they are on the premises, as when preparing tea or lunch in a staff restroom during a rest period.

Staff must not interfere with or misuse any health and safety equipment such as fire exits, fire extinguishers and warning notices. This includes any safety procedure applying to a kitchen, cloakroom or restroom.

How is the law enforced?

The Health and Safety at Work act is a criminal statute and the HSE is the enforcement body. Failure to carry out any duty under the Act is an offence and can lead to prosecution, a fine or even imprisonment. However, the HSE is firmly committed to persuasion; it has discretion to decide whether to prosecute and only does so after careful consideration. If a prosecution should occur, the courts will assess what is reasonably practicable in the light of available resources.

HSE inspectors have considerable powers. They may enter premises to enforce the law and do not need to seek permission before doing so (although they can enter only at a 'reasonable time'). They usually telephone to arrange a visit. Surprise inspections in response to an employer's complaint are rare. Otherwise, the usual reason for an unannounced visit is that an inspector has some spare time and includes a visit to a small premises within a schedule of visits to larger establishments. Although such visits may cause anxiety, this is not intended and the inspector should not be suspected of harbouring an ulterior motive.

If an inspector calls

If there are five or more staff, the inspector will want to see a statement of safety policy and instructions on safety procedures, and the accident book. He or she will examine the electrical equipment, which should be in good working order. Toilet and washing facilities should be at least equal to those required in offices. There should be hot and cold running water; the inspectors may propose wrist-operated taps in all rooms used for examining and treating patients. They will also be looking to ensure a practice has carried out a risk assessment as required under the new 'Management of Health and Safety' regulations.

What happens if the inspector is not satisfied?

When the inspection is completed, the inspector normally raises directly any improvements required. If these are not of major importance, he or she will simply ask that they are done as soon as possible. More serious matters could lead to a formal letter or even a written notice requiring them to be put right within a specified time. In these circumstances, the staff will be told of the inspector's intention to serve a written notice. In the unlikely event of a serious risk to health or safety, the inspector can issue a prohibition notice. Where there is a very serious risk, all work has to stop immediately.

The accident book

The employer is obliged to keep an accident book, in which all notifiable accidents and occurrences are recorded, so that these can be monitored and preventive action taken. Failure to do so could lead to a fine of up to £5000.

Violence to staff

Violence against GPs and their staff has been steadily increasing. The HSE wants to ensure that all employers take steps to protect their staff from violence. This is a corollary of the general obligation employers have to ensure the health and safety of their employees.

The health service advisory committee of the Health and Safety Commission has published advice in a booklet *Violence to Staff in the Health Service,* which emphasises the legal responsibilities of employers. It stresses that when violent incidents can be foreseen, employers have a duty to try to safeguard their staff. It advises against 'short, largely theoretical courses concerned with why violence and aggression occur': these will be insufficient to enable staff to develop the practical skills and confidence to handle violent patients.

The booklet also highlights areas where the risk of violence can be reduced:

- rearranging the seating and layout of waiting rooms;
- ensuring reception staff can keep an eye on patients and watch for signs of trouble (eg try to eliminate any blind corners in the waiting room);
- incorporating easy access or escape and alarms or panic buttons in treatment rooms;
- designing furniture and fittings so they cannot be used as weapons.

Particular attention should be paid to the risks of home visits by:

- keeping a record of staff whereabouts;
- setting up procedures for assessing potential or actual risk from patients;
- providing information on high-risk patients and practice areas.

All staff working in areas where there is a known high risk of violence should discuss its causes, learn to recognise signs of impending attack and develop the skills to deal with it. A plan should be drawn up so that staff are clear about what they should do in the event of a violent attack. They should be taught how to try to prevent the build-up of aggression in patients. They should also be forewarned against violent patients.

If there is a delay in surgery, explain this to patients. Try to defuse any incident. If all fails and confrontation seems inevitable, always back up your staff.

COSHH regulations

The Control of Substances Hazardous to Health Regulations 1968 (COSHH) impose additional obligations on employers. These apply to most hazardous substances except those covered by their own legislation, such as asbestos, lead and materials producing ionising radiation. The regulations set out the measures employers, the self-employed (and sometimes employees) have to take. Failure to comply exposes employees to risk and is an offence.

Hazardous substances include those labelled as dangerous (very toxic, toxic, harmful, irritant or corrosive) under the statutory requirements. The basic principles of occupational hygiene underlie the COSHH regulations. These include:

- assessing the risk to health arising from work and what precautions are needed;

- introducing measures to prevent or control the risk;

- ensuring control measures are used, equipment is properly maintained and procedures observed;

- monitoring, where necessary, the exposure of employees and carrying out an appropriate form of health surveillance;

- informing and training employees about the risks and precautions.

Other less dangerous substances covered by the regulations include disinfectants, clinical wastes, cleaning materials and, of course, drugs.

All employers should consider how COSHH regulations apply to their employees and working environment. Detailed information is available from the HSE.

An action list

- Issue a written statement of policy on health and safety to all staff, if there are five or more employees; this can be included in the employment contract;

- keep an accident book and a supply of copies of the accident report form;

- electrical equipment should be regularly maintained and serviced;

- an employee may be appointed as 'safety officer'; the practice manager may be most suited for this;

- known hazards should be regularly checked to see if any improvements are needed. Obvious examples include loose floor coverings, any building work, electrical plugs and equipment;

- patients and visitors should be warned by written notices of any hazards, particularly if there are building works in progress;

- the premises' lease or licence agreement should be reviewed; it should state who is responsible for maintaining and repairing the premises.

Looking to the Future

Sally Irvine

The introduction of the Charter for General Practice in the mid-1960s led to major changes in the delivery of primary care. Doctors were encouraged to form group practices, to improve their practice premises and to employ more ancillary staff in order to enlarge the range of their services. However, these services remained largely reactive and, for the resulting organisation to operate effectively, administrative skills were needed. Practice and health centre administrators came into existence. They were almost exclusively female and promoted from within the practice from senior receptionists and/or practice nurses. Many had been receptionists or secretaries only and most had no training for this role, which was seen as simply administrative. They were isolated from the wider world of the NHS.

Over the past 25 years this situation has changed – although fairly slowly – as preventive medicine, which needed planning skills, showed that the planned approach could be better than the reactive approach to the delivery of chronic and even acute care. Managing care became an obvious way of getting a handle on increased patient expectations and medical knowledge, as well as the technical implementation that was now possible. In addition, organisations such as the Association of Health Centre and Practice Administrators (AHCPA), the Association of Medical Secretaries and Practice Administrators and Receptionists (AMSPAR) and the Royal College of General Practitioners (RCGP), raised expectations both of doctors in management and of practice managers themselves.

Nevertheless, the role and function of management in practice has largely remained a Cinderella area with relatively low-paid non-medical managers, who have no clear definition of role, core content or competencies for the post of practice manager. It both attracts, and is frequently perceived to require, female postholders. This has ensured a continuing gender bias and a continuing inability of doctors to see the relevance to, and intrinsic partnership between, clinical care and non-clinical management. Practices that saw the need and value of the investment were few and far between.

The introduction of the new contract for general practitioners in 1990, and of fundholding in 1991, accelerated the process by recognising and clarifying the role of management as a new era in primary care was heralded. Greater and more diverse management skills are now needed to fulfil new responsibilities born of greater accountability. There has been an increase in the number of practice and fund managers recruited from outside and, as the remuneration has increased, many are now male.

It has also becoming increasingly clear that, to retain the general practitioner's role as the independent advocate of the patient, and the practice as the front-line of the health service, primary health care delivered from within general practice must be self-sufficient and manage its own quality. To that end, doctors themselves have had to acquire new management skills and a greater understanding of their role in the strategic driving seat not only of their practice, but of their neighbourhood as well. That has led to a greater involvement in, and understanding of, the nature and potential of medical and professional managers working together.

Moreover, district health authorities, family health service authorities and joint commissioning agencies are required to take a more strategic role in planning and developing primary health care services in the new 'managed' health service. For instance, traditional boundaries between primary care, secondary care, and the local population and local authorities are being redefined as multi-disciplinary teams prepare to meet the challenges presented by caring for people. The roles and responsibilities of the primary care teams are expanding as more and more GPs become fundholders and the team becomes more responsive to the health needs of its practice population.

This enhanced awareness and the opportunities and challenges it brings open up a number of areas of need for practice management. This chapter concentrates on four. These are:

- developing skills of development planning;

- responding to the training expectations of all members of the primary health care team as a fundamental part of management responsibility;

- establishing and agreeing to core competencies and standards for practice management to which all can respond;

- the management implications of 'purchasing' practices.

If practices can ensure these foundations are in place, it will help to ensure that general practice remains self-regulating, self-governing and independent. At the same time, it will demonstrate to doctors that they must overcome their inbred resistance to general management within practice.

Development planning

Every practice must now account in some way to its patients and to the taxpayer. The obvious way is through the annual practice report. The range of this document has extended as people realise that simply knowing what a practice has done without knowing what it intends to achieve is an arid exercise – hence the so-called business or development plan. For many practices, the value of planning ahead, of getting partners and staff to agree and be committed to common objectives and a programme of activity to achieve them, has been a goal for which they have striven for the benefit of the practice, not the FHSA. Sir Roy Griffiths summed it up: 'An effective management process needs personal accountability for performance against clear objectives, reasonably precise resources, and a clear timescale for performance'.

Strategic planning is all about looking ahead and much of the value of a development plan lies in answering the key questions:

- Why is the organisation here?

- What business is it in?

- What are its politics?

- What does it intend to do to enact that purpose?

Answering these questions takes time, commitment and a leader, be it the senior partner or the practice manager. That leader must be someone who understands the process itself and can enable others to articulate their own agendas and translate thoughts into coherent statements. The central role of the person managing the practice is to stimulate, to initiate and even to bully their way to a consensus statement or plan that has agreed action attached to it. This sort of management role is vital if development planning is to achieve its potential to underpin clinical care.

Fundholding cannot exist without proper planned development, not because fundholding practices are money-oriented but because, if they are to be responsible for the resources that are needed, they must be planned, consistent, organised and disciplined in their approach.

So do those who claim a role as advocates of patients. All practices need to know whether they are achieving what they said they would achieve, and the results can give a tremendous boost to practice confidence. A plan can focus on fact and not opinion. It can develop teamwork and a team approach, and above all it can identify the skills area within the team. This leads to the next major area of development in the future for practice management, training.

Training

Training and development within non-clinical areas, particularly in general practice, have a low profile within the prevailing culture, which places a much greater emphasis on direct patient care. Training opportunities are typically designed for groups from a single profession, and although teamwork is a widely articulated goal, structural and attitudinal barriers make it difficult to sustain and develop in the training field. It is vital that the practice manager within the team and within his or her own profession responds to the challenge of both the training itself and the context in which it operates. The practice must see and sell training as an investment which, by providing the organisation with the right people at the right time and with the right skills, must contribute to achieving its strategic objectives. At the same time, people who are encouraged to go on learning and developing throughout their working lives will be better motivated and better able to contribute to the success of their organisation.

There is a fundamental link between the organisation's objectives set out in the development plan, the first major area of challenge described above, and the training and development undertaken by those delivering the plan, to ensure that there are appropriate resources to deliver it. The management of the practice needs to be fully aware and have access to information about what training is available, where and from whom.

In devising a training programme alongside the development plan, not only are skills and needs identified but they should be monitored and developed after training. Appropriate funding is needed both from within the practice and from outside agencies. Knowing how to get this funding is a vital role for the practice manager.

In addition, practice managers need to provide in-house 'modelling' as well as training for all members of the team (including the medical members). This role must not be underestimated. However, practice managers need time for their own training. To identify their needs assumes an agreed 'bag' of competencies and standards for their professionalism. This brings us to the next major challenge for practice management.

Standards

The development of nationally accepted standards for managers in general practice is vital. Postholders need to have a clear, marketable and professional basis for their development, particularly to empower the non-medical female members of the practice team. With this goes the need to define the role of practice managers and their relationship within the new accredited qualifications through NCVQ Levels 1-4 and the Management Charter Initiatives (MCI) 1 and 2. There is a need to identify clear and unequivocal benchmarks or standards of competence which provide a basis against which practice management can be assessed, performance improved and skills more effectively utilised. The competencies identified should be based on what managers actually do, an agreement of what effective management performance within general practice is, and the level of performance that employers can expect. Practices which have been involved in audit, quality assurance and the acquisition of BS 5750 are already on the way to identifying such standards.

Management standards should reflect the management needs of the practice, whether managers are medical or non-medical. It is this concept of partnership within the management of the practice that is one of the biggest challenges in providing clear, nationally agreed standards.

The role of both medical and non-medical professional associations is vital in defining and educating for particular standards. Organisations such as AHCPA and the RCGP must work together to produce a strong and secure base to prevent external management within the health service taking responsibility for the quality both of medical work and the management within general practices.

Purchasing – the individual or the practice

The final area describes the biggest challenge of all, one that derives directly from the new reforms and the new market economy and the new buzz phrase, the 'purchaser/provider split'. Whoever invented that phrase could have made a fortune in royalties!

Practices are increasingly having a powerful influence on the quality of care through the contracting process, either directly in the case of services which fundholders purchase or indirectly for all practices through the commissioning strategies of district health authorities.

The biggest challenge to management remains the managing of a service where the employers are also the floor-workers. Practice-based provision (and therefore contracts) may well be the way forward, with the individual contractor a thing of the past. For managers, this presents a range of problems, from clinical compliance to real teamwork, and a range of activities which, while not new, will have a sharper edge. As cost-containment begins to bite, there will have to be tighter monitoring of individual clinicians' performance within the practice. Managing conflict will be another skill to be learned!

Conclusion

The four areas described above are not the only challenges for the future but they seem to be the most exciting and demanding. The clock cannot be turned back: the new style and approach to health care and its rationing are here to stay. The opportunity lies in managing the balance between the discipline of rationing and the indiscipline of caring, and doing so in a way that retains satisfaction for the professionals, meets the expectations of the public and stays within budgets. For managers in practice, this must be a challenge worth meeting.

Part Six

Directory of Products, Services and Suppliers to the Health Care Industry

Directory of Products, Services and Suppliers to the Health Care Industry

Acupuncture teaching

Complementary medical practices   –   courses
                                              –   seasonal affective disorder

Conference and exhibition centres and organisers

Dietary management and vitamin supplements

Health promotion

Hospital group (private)

Incontinence supplies

Inter-medical services

Laboratory services

Laboratory services   –   nutrition and environmental

Magnetic resonance imaging

Medical and dental indemnity organisations

Medical equipment and sundries   –   dressings and bandages
                                              –   medical equipment
                                              –   protective clothing and gloves
                                              –   specialist implants and prostheses
                                              –   sterilising equipment

Medical insurance

Medical products

Medical publications

Mental health

Office equipment
- communications systems
- dictionaries and directories
- furniture, furnishings and secure storage
- information systems
- stationery

Patient services
- facilities and treatment

Property services

Security
- consultancy, equipment and systems

Services and consultancy
- contract car hire and leasing
- financial
- legal
- management, marketing and PR
- pharmaceutical selling
- training and recruitment
- travel health
- video services

Skin clinic
- tattoo removal

Specialist patient care/treatment

Waste management

Acupuncture teaching

British College of Acupuncture
8 Hunter Street
London WC1 1BN
Tel: 071 833 8164

Complementary medical practice – courses

BIOLAB Medical Unit
9 Weymouth Street
London W1N 3FF
Tel: 071 580 3526

The British College of Acupuncture
8 Hunter Street
London WC1N 1BN
Tel: 071 833 8164

The British School of Osteopathy
1–4 Suffolk Street
London SW1Y 4HG
Tel: 071 930 9254

The Dallamore College of Advanced Reflexology
50 Sidney Dye Court
Sporle, Kings Lynn
Norfolk PE32 2EE
Tel: 0760 725437

David Lewis Centre
Mill Lane
Warford
Near Alderley Edge
Cheshire SK9 7UD
Tel: 0565 872613

The Institute of Counselling
15 Hope Street
Glasgow G2 6AE
Tel: 041 204 2230

The Proudfoot School of Hypnosis and Psychotherapy
9 Belvedere Place
Scarborough
North Yorkshire YO11 2QN
Tel: 0723 363638

Regent's College
School of Psychotherapy and
Counselling
Inner Circle
Regent's Park
London NW1 4NS
Tel: 071 487 7406

School of Meditation
158 Holland Park Avenue
London W11 4UH
Tel: 071 437 0097

The School of Phytotherapy
Bucksteep Manor
Bodle Street Green
Hailsham
East Sussex BN27 4RJ
Tel: 0323 833812/4

Stop Smoking
PO Box 100
Plymouth
Devon PL1 1RG
Tel: 0752 709506

Complementary medical practice – seasonal affective disorder

Outside In
Unit 5, Dry Drayton Industries
Scotland Road
Dry Drayton
Cambridge CB2 1BR
Tel: 0934 211955

Conference and exhibition centres and organisers

Aberdeen Exhibition and Conference Centre
Bridge of Don, Aberdeen
Grampian AB2 8BL
Tel: 0224 824824

Abbey Park Hotel
The Mount
York YO2 2BA
Tel: 0904 65801

Barbican Centre
Barbican
London EC2Y 8DS
Tel: 071 638 4141

Bournemouth International Centre
Exeter Road, Bournemouth
Dorset BH2 5BH
Tel: 0202 552122

Brighton Centre
Brighton Conference Office
Marlborough House
54 Old Steine
Brighton
East Sussex BN1 1EQ
Tel: 0273 21173

Business Design Centre
52 Upper Street, Islington
London N1 0QH
Tel: 071 359 3535

Earls Court Exhibition Centre
Warwick Road
London SW5 9TA
Tel: 071 385 1200

EMAP International Exhibitions
12 Bedford Row
London WC1R 4DU
Tel: 071 404 4844

Evan Steadman Group
The Hub, 9 Emson Close
Saffron Waldon
Essex CB10 1HL
Tel: 0799 26699

Event Presentations Ltd
Petworth Road
Witley, Godalming
Surrey GU8 5QW
Tel: 0483 426608

Fairfield Halls
Park Lane
Croydon
Surrey CR9 1DG
Tel: 081 681 0821

Fairs and Exhibitions Ltd
Suite 12, Accurist House
Baker Street
London W1M 2HH
Tel: 071 935 8537

G-Mex Centre
The Greater Manchester Exhibition
and Event Centre
City Centre
Manchester M2 3GX
Tel: 061 834 2700

The Hexagon
Queens Walk
Reading
Berkshire RG1 7UA
Fax: 0734 487434

Naidex Conventions Ltd
90 Calverley Road
Tunbridge Wells
Kent TN1 2UN
Tel: 0892 544027

National Exhibition Centre Ltd
Exhibitions Division
Birmingham B40 1NT
Tel: 021 780 4171

Octagon Centre
University of Sheffield
Western Bank
Sheffield S10 2TQ
Tel: 0742 768555

Olympia Conference Centre
Olympia 2, Kensington
Hammersmith Road
London W14 8UX
Tel: 071 603 8067

Park Hotels
26 Queens Garden
London W2 3BD
Tel: 071 262 0222/723 4737

The Queen Elizabeth II Conference Centre
Broad Sanctuary, Westminster
London SW1P 3EE
Tel: 071 798 4060

Reed Exhibitions Group
Oriel House
26 The Quadrant
Richmond upon Thames
Surrey TW9 1DL
Tel: 081 940 6065

The Town Hall, Kensington
Royal Borough of Kensington and
Chelsea
Hornton Street
London W8 7NX
Tel: 071 937 5464

Dietary management and vitamin supplements

BIOLAB Medical Unit
9 Weymouth Street
London W1N 3FF
Tel: 071 580 3526

Kimal Scientific Products Ltd
Arundel Road Industrial Estate
Uxbridge
Middlesex UB8 2SA
Tel: 0895 70951

Lamberts Healthcare Ltd
1 Lamberts Road
Tunbridge Wells
Kent TN2 3EQ
Tel: 0892 534574

G R Lane Health Products
Sisson Road
Gloucester GL1 3QB
Tel: 0452 524012

Napp Laboratories
Cambridge Science Park
Milton Road
Cambridge CB4 4GW
Tel: 0223 424444

Surgicon Ltd
84 Wakefield Road
Brighouse
West Yorkshire HD6 1QL
Tel: 0484 712147

Weight Watchers (UK) Ltd
Kidwells Park House
Kidwells Park Drive
Maidenhead
Berkshire SL6 8YT
Tel: 0628 777077

York Nutritional Laboratory
Tudor House, Lysander Close
Clifton Moor
York YO3 4XB
Tel: 0904 690640

Health promotion

Stop Smoking
PO Box 100
Plymouth
Devon PL1 1RG
Tel: 0752 709506

Hospital group (private)

BMI Healthcare
4 Cornwall Terrace
Regents Park
London NW1 4QP
Tel: 071 486 1266

Incontinence supplies

Deputy Healthcare
Millshaw House
Manor Mill Lane
Leeds LS11 8LQ
Tel: 0532 706000

Inter-medical services

British Airways Travel Clinics
7 Bury Place
London WC1A 2LA
Tel: 071 831 3266

Cedar Falls Health Farm
Bishops Lydeard
Taunton
Somerset TA4 3HR
Tel: 0823 433233

Central Sheffield University Hospitals
Royal Hallamshire Hospital
Glossop Road
Sheffield S10 2JF
Tel: 0742 766222 ext 3456

Clouds House
East Knoyle
Wiltshire SP3 6BE
Tel: 0747 830733

Community Hospitals Ltd
Priory Terrace
Bromham Road
Bedford MK40 2QD
Tel: 0234 273473

Cytogenetic Services
48 Wimpole Street
London W1M 7DG
Tel: 071 486 1322

Cytoserve Ltd
Landsdowne House
63 Balby Road
Doncaster DN4 0RE
Tel: 0302 730316

The David Lewis Centre
Mill Lane
Warford, nr Alderley Edge
Cheshire SK9 7UD
Tel: 0565 872613

The Devonshire Hospital
29–31 Devonshire Street
London W1N 1RF
Tel: 071 486 7131

Dewsbury District Hospital
Healds Road
Dewsbury
West Yorkshire WF13 4HS
Tel: 0924 455736

Glenfield General Hospital
Groby Road
Leicester LE3 9QP
Tel: 0533 871471

Harley Street Sports Clinic
110 Harley Street
London W1
Tel: 071 486 2494

Huntercombe Manor
Huntercombe Lane South
Taplow
Berkshire SL6 0PQ
Tel: 0628 667881

The London Clinic
20 Devonshire Place
London W1H 2DH
Tel: 071 935 4444

LCPC (London Clinical Pathology Consultants) Ltd
19 Wimpole Street
London W1M 7AD
Tel: 071 436 1930

The Manor House Hospital
North End Road
Golders Green
London NW11 7HX
Tel: 081 455 6601

The Maudsley Hospital
Denmark Hill
London SE5 8AZ
Tel: 071 703 6333

Mount Vernon Hospital
Rickmansworth Road
Northwood
Middlesex HA6 2RN
Tel: 0895 278250

Queen Square Imaging Centre
8–11 Queen Square
London WC1N 3AR
Tel: 071 833 2513

Riverside Health Authority
Westminster Hospital
Dean Ryle Street
London SW1P 2AP
Tel: 081 746 8234

St Anthony's Hospital
London Road
North Cheam
Surrey SM3 9DW
Tel: 081 337 6691

St James' University Hospital
Beckett Street
Leeds LS9 7TF
Tel: 0532 433144

St Thomas' Hospital
London SE1 7EH
Tel: 071 928 9292

Sutton's Manor Clinic
London Road
Stapleford Tawney
Essex RM4 1SR
Tel: 0992 814661

Thomson Cytology Services
6 London Street
London W2 1HR
Tel: 071 258 3940

Ward Surgical Services
Bensham House
325–340 Bensham Lane
Thornton Heath
London CR7 7EQ
Tel: 081 684 0470

The Woodbourne Clinic
21 Woodbourne Road
Birmingham B17 8BY
Tel: 021 434 4343

York Nutritional Laboratory
Tudor House, Lysander Close
Clifton Moor
York YO3 4XB
Tel: 0904 690640

The Yorkshire Clinic
Bradford Road
Bingley
West Yorkshire BD16 1TW
Tel: 0274 560311

Laboratory services

Medi-Lab Ltd
The Regency Hospital
Macclesfield SK11 8DW
Tel: 0625 501801

Sheffield Pathology Services
Northern General Hospital
Herries Road
Sheffield S5 7AU
Tel: 0742 562954

Laboratory services – nutrition and environmental

BIOLAB Medical Unit
9 Weymouth Street
London W1N 3FF
Tel: 071 580 3526

Magnetic resonance imaging

Queen Square Imaging Centre
8–11 Queen Square
London WC1N 3AR
Tel: 071 833 2513

Medical and dental indemnity organisations

The Medical Protection Society
50 Hallam Street
London W1N 6DE
Tel: 071 637 0541

Medical equipment and sundries – dressings and bandages

Aremco
Grove House
Lenham
Kent ME17 2PX
Tel: 0622 858502

Convatec
Harrington House
Milton Road
Ickenham
Middlesex UB10 8PU
Tel: 0895 678888

Cory Bros Ltd
4 Dollis Park
Finchley
London N3 1HG
Tel: 081 349 1081

DRG Hospital Supplies Ltd
1 Dixon Road
Brislington
Bristol BS4 5BY
Tel: 0272 716111

Johnson and Johnson Medical Ltd
Coronation Road
Ascot
Berkshire SL5 9EY
Tel: 0344 872626

Kirton Healthcare Group Ltd
Bungay Road, Hempnall
Norwich NR15 2NG
Tel: 050842 8411

Mediflex Ltd
Unit 20, Broombank Business Park
Broombank Road
Sheepbridge
Chesterfield S41 9QJ
Tel: 0246 455928

Relyon Ltd
PO Box 1, Wellington
Somerset TA21 8NN
Tel: 0823 667501

Robinson Health Care
Hipper House
Chesterfield S40 1YF
Tel: 0246 220022

John Scarborough and Partners Ltd
Orchard House
West Bradley, nr Glastonbury
Somerset BA6 8PB
Tel: 0458 50491

Seton Healthcare International plc
Tubiton House, Brook Street
Oldham OL1 3HS
Tel: 061 652 2222

Smith and Nephew Medical Ltd
Brierfield Mills
Brierfield, Nelson
Lancashire BB9 5NJ
Tel: 0280 67744

Steriseal
Thornhill Road
Redditch
Worcestershire B98 9NL
Tel: 0527 64222

Surgicon Ltd
84 Wakefield Road
Brighouse
West Yorkshire HD6 1QL
Tel: 0484 712147

3M Health Care Ltd
3M House
Morley Street
Loughborough
Leicestershire LE11 1EP
Tel: 0509 611611

Medical equipment and sundries – medical equipment

AFP Medical
Unit 71, Somers Road
Rugby
Warwickshire CV22 7DG
Tel: 0788 579408

Air-Shields Vickers
Cranbourne House
Bessemer Road
Basingstoke
Hampshire RG21 3NB
Tel: 0256 29141

APC Cardiovascular Ltd
18 Macon Court
Macon Way
Crewe
Cheshire DW1 1EA
Tel: 0270 216142

Becton Dickinson UK Ltd
Between Towns Road
Cowley
Oxford OX4 3LY
Tel: 0865 777722

Biomen Diagnostic Division
Tripod House
105–107 Lansdowne Road
Croydon
Surrey CR0 2BN
Tel: 081 681 5679

Bodystat Ltd
16 Mount Havelock
Douglas
Isle of Man
Tel: 0642 28571

Braun and Co Ltd
19 Pasture Road
Barton on Humber
South Humberside DN18 5HN
Tel: 0652 33399

Cardiokinetics Ltd
2 Kansas Avenue
Salford M5 2GL
Tel: 061 872 8287

Cranlea and Co
The Sandpits
Acacia Road
Bourneville
Birmingham B30 2AH
Tel: 021 482 0361

Ellisons
Crondal Road
Exhall
Coventry CV7 9NH
Tel: 0203 36169

Graseby Medical Ltd
Colonial Way
Watford
Hertfordshire WD2 4LG
Tel: 0923 246434

Gulfex Medical and Scientific Ltd
7 Burgess Wood Road South
Beaconsfield
Buckinghamshire HP9 1EU
Tel: 0494 675353

Hawksley and Sons Ltd
Marlborough Road
Lancing
West Sussex BN15 8TN
Tel: 0903 752815

Healthguard (UK) Ltd
Unit 12, Danesbury Rise
Cheadle
Cheshire SK8 1JW
Tel: 061 428 5413

Inner Resources
Lesley Road
Woodford Park Industrial Estate
Winford
Cheshire CN7 2SP
Tel: 0606 853554/86137

Kontron Instruments Ltd
Blackmoor Lane
Croxley Centre
Watford
Hertfordshire WD1 8XQ
Tel: 0923 56252

Ohmeda
Ohmeda House
71 Great North Road
Hatfield
Hertfordshire AL9 5EN
Tel: 0707 263570

Omron Healthcare GMBH
c/o Hutchings Healthcare Ltd
Rede House
New Barn Lane
Henfield
West Sussex BN5 9SJ
Tel: 0273 490533

Owen Mumford Ltd
Medical Division
Brook Hill
Woodstock
Oxford OX20 1TU
Tel: 0993 812921

Oxford Medical Ltd
1 Kimber Road
Abingdon
Oxfordshire OX14 1BZ
Tel: 0235 533433

Reynolds Medical Ltd
Cawthorne House
51 St Andrew's Street
Hertford SG14 1HZ
Tel: 0992 558211

Seward Medical Ltd
131 Great Suffolk Street
London SE1 1PP
Tel: 071 357 6727

3M Health Care Ltd
3M House
Morley Street
Loughborough
Leicestershire LE11 1EP
Tel: 0509 611611

Medical equipment and sundries – protective clothing and gloves

Alexandra Workwear plc
Alexandra House
Britannia Road
Patchway
Bristol BS12 5TP
Tel: 0272 690808

DRG Hospital Supplies Ltd
1 Dixon Road
Brislington
Bristol BS4 5BY
Tel: 0272 716111

Lojigma International Ltd
Elgin Industrial Estate
Dunfermline, Scotland
Tel: 0383 730156

Mediflex Ltd
Unit 20, Broombank Business Park
Broombank Road
Sheepbridge
Chesterfield S41 9QJ
Tel: 0246 455928

Nurse-Care Uniform Co Ltd
11 Lime Street
Southampton SO1 1DA
Tel: 0703 225335

Regent Hospital Products
LRC Products Ltd
North Circular Road
London E4 8QA
Tel: 081 527 2377

Spentex BCA Ltd
Street 7
Thorp Arch Trading Estate
Wetherby
West Yorkshire LS23 7BJ
Tel: 0937 845429

Vernon-Carus Ltd
Penwortham Mills
Penwortham
Preston PR1 9SN
Tel: 0772 744493

L Wells (London) Ltd
PO Box 35, Guildford
Surrey GU4 8AH
Tel: 0483 572236

The Westbrook Linen Co Ltd
Northbeck Mills
PO Box 16, Keighley
West Yorkshire BD21 1RZ
Tel: 0535 667625

Medical equipment and sundries – specialist implants and prostheses

Royal National Orthopaedic Hospital Trust
Brockley Hill
Stanmore
Middlesex HA7 4LP
Tel: 081 954 2300

Medical equipment and sundries – sterilising equipment

Atesmo Contracting Service Ltd
Unit 7
Tyndall Street Industrial Estate
Cardiff CF1 5BG
Tel: 0222 488800/484567

BMM Weston Ltd
Weston Works
Faversham
Kent ME13 7EB
Tel: 0795 532246

Harvard/LTE
Greenbridge Lane
Greenfield
Oldham OL3 7EN
Tel: 0457 876221

Janssen Pharmaceutical Ltd
Grove
Wantage
Oxon OX12 0DQ
Tel: 0235 777333

Kestrel
115 Oldham Road
Rochdale OL16 5QT
Tel: 0706 47499

Keymed
Keymed House
Stock Road
Southend on Sea
Essex SS2 5QH
Tel: 0702 616333

Medical Installations Co Ltd
Wilbraham Road
Fulbourn
Cambridge CB1 5ET
Tel: 0223 880909

The Sterilizing Equipment Co Ltd
Kings Mill Way
Hermitage Lane Industrial Estate
Mansfield NG18 5ER
Tel: 0623 646841

3M Health Care Ltd
3M House
Morley Street
Loughborough
Leicestershire LE11 1EP
Tel: 0509 611611

Medical insurance

Nationwide Physiotherapy Service
The Manor House
Squires Hill
Rothwell
Northamptonshire NN14 2BQ
Tel: 0536 713713

Medical products

Astra Pharmaceuticals
Home Park
Kings Langley
Hertfordshire WD4 8DH
Tel: 0923 266191

Bayer UK Ltd
Bayer House
Strawberry Hill
Newbury
Berkshire RG13 1JA
Tel: 0635 39000

David Lewis Centre
Mill Lane
Warford
Near Alderley Edge
Cheshire SK9 7UD
Tel: 0565 872613

Depuy Healthcare
Millshaw House
Manor Mill Lane
Leeds LS11 8LQ
Tel: 0532 706000

Elida Gibbs Ltd
Hesketh House
Portman Square
London W1A 1DY
Tel: 071 486 1200

Janssen Pharmaceuticals
Grove
Wantage
Oxfordshire OX12 0DQ
Tel: 0235 772966

London International Group
35 New Bridge Street
London EC4
Tel: 071 489 1977

Owen Mumford Ltd
Brook Hill
Woodstock
Oxon OX20 1TU
Tel: 0992 812021

Pharmax Ltd
Bourne End
Bexley
Kent DA5 1NX
Tel: 0322 550550

Trident (UK) Ltd
21 Grove Road
Havant
Hampshire PO9 1AR
Tel: 0705 475901

The Wellcome Foundation Ltd
PO Box 129
160 Euston Road
London NW1 2BP
Tel: 071 387 4477

Medical publications

British Journal of General Practice
12 Queen Street
Edinburgh EH2 1JE
Tel: 031 225 7629

BMA News Review
BMA House
Tavistock Square
London WC1H 9JP
Tel: 071 387 4499

British Medical Journal
BMA House
Tavistock Square
London WC1H 9JP
Tel: 071 387 4499

David Lewis Centre
Mill Lane
Warford
Near Alderley Edge
Cheshire SK9 7UD
Tel: 0565 872613

Doctor
Quadrant House
The Quadrant
Sutton
Surrey SM2 5AS
Tel: 081 661 8740

General Practitioner
Haymarket Publishing
30 Lancaster Gate
London W2 3LP
Tel: 081 943 5000

Lancet
42 Bedford Square
London WC1B 3SL
Tel: 071 436 4981

Medeconomics
30 Calderwood Street
Woolwich
London SE18 6QH
Tel: 081 855 7777

Practice Manager
Reed Healthcare Communications
Quadrant House
The Quadrant
Sutton
Surrey SM2 5AS
Tel: 081 661 3500

Response Marketing 'Nationwide' Ltd
3 All Hallows Road
Bispham
Blackpool FY2 0AF
Tel: 0253 500860

Scottish Medical Journal
Department of Medicine
Ninewells Hospital and Medical School
Dundee DD1 9SY
Tel: 0382 60111

Mental health

The Maudsley
The Maudsley Hospital
Denmark Hill
London SE5 8AZ
Tel: 071 703 6333

Office equipment – communications systems

Contacta Communication Systems Ltd
Imex House, VIP Trading Estate
Anchor and Hope Lane
London SE7 7TE
Tel: 081 8588 2123

Contarnex Ltd
252 Martin Way
Morden
Surrey SM4 4AW
Tel: 081 540 1034

Dictaphone Co Ltd
Regent Square House
The Parade, Leamington Spa
Warwickshire CV32 4NL
Tel: 0926 451155

Medical Installations Co Ltd
Wilbraham Road, Fulbourn
Cambridge CB1 5ET
Tel: 0223 880909

Mercury Communications Ltd
New Mercury House
26 Red Lion Square
London WC1R 4HQ
Tel: 071 528 2000

Philips Business Systems
Elektra House
2 Bergholt Road
Colchester
Essex CO4 5BE
Tel: 0206 575115

Ritel Communication Freedom
Marshgate Trading Estate
Stratton Road
Swindon SN1 2PA
Tel: 0793 616166

RPL Telecommunications plc
19 The Metropolitan Centre
Derby Road, Greenford
Middlesex
Tel: 081 575 9999

Thorn EMI Business Communications
8 Roxborough Way
Foundation Park, Maidenhead
Berkshire SL6 2BE
Tel: 0628 822181

Office equipment – dictionaries and directories

Bumpus Haldane and Maxwell
4 Midland Road
Olney
Buckinghamshire MK46 4BN
Tel: 0234 711529

Butterworth-Heinemann
PO Box 63, Westbury House
Guildford
Surrey GU2 5BH
Tel: 0483 300066

Croner Publications Ltd
Croner House, London Road
Kingston upon Thames KT2 6SR
Tel: 081 547 3333

Dillons Bookstore
82 Gower Street
London WC1E 6EQ
Tel: 071 636 1577

Gower Publishing Co
Gower House, Croft Road
Aldershot
Hampshire GU11 3HR
Tel: 0252 331551

Kogan Page Ltd
120 Pentonville Road
London N1 9JN
Tel: 071 278 0433

Laing and Buisson
111B Regent's Park Road
London NW1 8UR
Tel: 071 722 9272

Scutari Projects Ltd
Viking House
17–19 Peterborough Road
Harrow
Middlesex HA1 2AX
Tel: 081 423 1066

STM Books
561 Watford Way
Mill Hill
London NW7 3JR
Tel: 081 959 0144

**Office equipment – furniture,
furnishings and secure storage**

Antocks Lairn Ltd
Lancaster Road
Cressex, High Wycombe
Buckinghamshire HP12 3HX
Tel: 0494 465454

The Back Shop
24 New Cavendish Street
London W1
Tel: 071 935 9148

Will Beck Ltd
Kitchener Chair Works
Kitchener Road
High Wycombe
Buckinghamshire HP11 2SW
Tel: 0494 524466

Byrum UK Ltd
Milton Hall
Milton, Cambridge
Tel: 0223 440833

Richard Craven and Co Ltd
Manse Lane
Knaresborough
North Yorkshire HG5 8ET
Tel: 0423 869111

Ercol Furniture
London Road
High Wycombe
Buckinghamshire HP13 7AE
Tel: 0494 21261

Flexiform
The Office Furniture Centre
1392 Leeds Road
Bradford
West Yorkshire BD3 7AE
Tel: 0274 656013

GLS Fairway
Ferry Lane, Tottenham Hale
London N17 9QN
Tel: 081 801 3333

George Hinchliffe Ltd
104–106 King Street
Dukinfield
Cheshire SK16 4LJ
Tel: 061 330 1008/2198

Heckmondwike FB Ltd
PO Box 7
Wellington Mills, Liversedge
West Yorkshire WF15 7XA
Tel: 0924 406161

Hoskins Ltd
Upper Trinity Street
Birmingham B9 4EQ
Tel: 021 766 7404

Lamson Industries (UK) Ltd
Oak House
Clayton Avenue, Hassocks
West Sussex BN6 8BH
Tel: 0273 844310

Lister and Co plc
Manningham Mills
Bradford
West Yorkshire BD9 4SH
Tel: 0274 542222

Peter Moreton and Sons Ltd
Whitacre Road
Nuneaton
Warwickshire
Tel: 0203 384841/347578

New Concept Treatment Couches
Cox Hall Lane
Tattingstone
Ipswich IP9 2NS
Tel: 0473 328006

Project Office Furniture plc
Hamlet Green
Haverhill
Suffolk CB9 8QJ
Tel: 0440 705411

Portasilo Ltd
Huntington
York YO3 9PR
Tel: 0904 624872

Rhondeau
Unit 4, George Bayliss Road
Berry Hill Industrial Estate
Droitwich
Worcestershire WR9 9AB
Tel: 0905 773300

Office equipment – information systems

Applied Medical Technology Ltd
1 Orwell Furlong, Cowley Road
Cambridge CB4 4WY
Tel: 0223 420415

The Computer Centre
Maskew Avenue
Peterborough PE1 2AQ
Tel: 0733 558919

Horizon Software Ltd
27 East Street
Leicester LE1 6NB
Tel: 0533 556550

Hoskyns Group plc
130 Shaftesbury Avenue
London W1V 7DN
Tel: 071 434 2171

IBM (UK) Ltd
PO Box 41, North Harbour
Portsmouth PO6 3AU
Tel: 0705 321212

ICL (UK) Ltd
ICL House, Putney
London SW15 1SW
Tel: 081 788 7272
also at
Computer House, 127 Hagley Road
Edgbaston
Birmingham B16 8LD
Tel: 021 456 1111
and
Arndale House
Manchester M4 3AR
Tel: 061 833 9111

Intac Data Systems Ltd
Surrey House, Morthern Road
Thurcroft, Rotherham
South Yorkshire S66 9JG
Tel: 0709 547177

Logic Information Systems
191 Shoreditch High Street
London E1 6HU
Tel: 071 739 2941

Meduser Systems Ltd
Kingsnorth House
Wotton Road
Ashford
Kent TN23 2LN
Tel: 1233 622335

Online Information Services Ltd
152 Main Road
Long Hanborough
Oxford OX7 2MD
Tel: 0423 884805

Philips Information Systems
Elektra House
2 Bergholt Road
Colchester
Essex CO4 5BE
Tel: 0206 575115

Office equipment – stationery

Budget Direct Ltd
Global House
38–40 High Street
West Wickham
Kent BR4 0NE
Tel: 081 777 0099

Hill International Ltd
Hill House
45–53 George Street
Newcastle upon Tyne NE4 7LQ
Tel: 091 273 9261

Mastrom Ltd
Alrewas
Burton on Trent
Staffordshire DE13 7AG
Tel: 0283 790030

Parker Pen UK Ltd
Newhaven
East Sussex BN9 0AU
Tel: 0273 513233

Wespac Ltd
154–8 Shoreditch High Street
London E1 6HU
Tel: 071 415 9000

Patient services – facilities and treatment

The London Clinic
20 Devonshire Place
London W1N 2DH
Tel: 071 935 4444

Property services

Architects Co-Partnership
Northaw House
Potters Bar
Hertfordshire EN6 4PS
Tel: 0707 51141

Charles-Jones Park and Miers, Architects
483 Liverpool Road
London N7 8PG
Tel: 071 607 6412

EP Associates
3 Stukeley Street
London WC2
Tel: 071 831 4464

EPR Architects Ltd
21 Douglas Street
London SW1P 4PE
Tel: 071 834 4411

Health Care Buildings Ltd
36 Paradise Road
Richmond
Surrey TW9 1SE
Tel: 081 948 5544

Hedlunds Swedish Houses Ltd
Hedlunds House
Beacon Road
Crowborough
Sussex TN6 1AF
Tel: 0892 665007

Llewelyn-Davies Weeks
Brook House
2–16 Torrington Place
London WC1E 7HN
Tel: 071 637 0181

Portakabin Ltd
Huntington
York YO3 9PT
Tel: 0904 611655

Spooner Accommodation Ltd
Main Road, Wyton
Hull HU11 4DJ
Tel: 0482 815341

Graham G Stephens and Partners
62 College Road, Maidstone
Kent ME15 6SJ
Tel: 0622 751969

Welconstruct Co Ltd
127 Hagley Road
Birmingham B16 8XU
Tel: 021 455 9798

Security – consultancy, equipment and systems

Ambassador Security Group
Hermitage Court
Hermitage Lane
Barming, Maidstone
Kent ME16 9NT
Tel: 0622 720780

Borer Data Systems Ltd
6 Market Place
Wokingham
Berkshire RG11 1AL
Tel: 0734 791137

Cam Era Holdings
Kembury House
5 Worcester Road
Bromsgrove B61 7DL
Tel: 0527 579669

Case-Cash and Security Equipment Ltd
Security House
Acrewood Way
St Albans
Hertfordshire AL4 0JL
Tel: 0727 868203

Coralplan
27A Elizabeth Mews
London NW3 4UH
Tel: 071 483 0350

Crownpound Ltd
Unit 7, Mill Farm Business Park
Millfield Road
Hanworth
Middlesex TW4 5PY
Tel: 081 893 3757

Selectamark Security Systems Ltd
10 Plaistow Lane
Bromley
Kent BR1 3PA
Tel: 081 464 0414

Smiths Security Services
111 Walton Street
Oxford OX2 6AJ
Tel: 0865 57454

Thorn Home Security
Central Park
Ohio Avenue
Salford M5 2GT
Tel: 061 876 7235

Services and consultancy – contract car hire and leasing

The Association of Car Fleet Operators
1 The Hermitage
Richmond
Surrey TW10 6SH
Tel: 081 940 1692

Auto Contracts
10 Albert Drive
Glasgow G41
Tel: 041 424 4141
also at
12 West Mayfield
Edinburgh EH9 1TG
Tel: 031 662 4646

BRS Car Lease
Imperial House
Holly Walk, Leamington Spa
Warwickshire CV32 4YB
Tel: 0926 450100

Carline
77 Mortlake High Street
London SW14 8HL
Tel: 081 878 8617

Fleet Motor Management Ltd
Eaton Ford, St Neots
Cambridgeshire PE19 4AG
Tel: 0480 75757

Leasecontracts plc
Lauriston House
Pitchill, Evesham
Worcestershire WR11 5SN
Tel: 0386 870884

Meashams of Greenford
Greenford Road
Greenford
Middlesex UB6 8RE
Tel: 081 578 2633

Robins and Day
9th Floor, Trafford House
Chester Road
Manchester M32 0RS
Tel: 061 873 7618
also at
Noble House
143 Hersham Road
Walton on Thames
Surrey KT12 1RR
Tel: 0932 246664
and
Clock House
Newport Road
Castle Bromwich
Birmingham B36 8BQ
Tel: 021 749 6000/706 5808

Services and consultancy – financial

Abbey National Financial Services
Knights Templar House
38–42 Frogmoor
High Wycombe
Buckinghamshire HP13 5DH
Tel: 0494 472211

Allied Dunbar Assurance plc
Allied Dunbar Centre
Swindon SN1 1EL
Tel: 0793 514514

The Bank of Scotland
Marketing Department
Uberior House, 61 Grassmarket
Edinburgh EH1 2JF
Tel: 0800 838113

Barclays Information Centre
Department TM
Freepost
Northampton NN1 1BR
Tel: 0800 400170

Benson and Co
The Old Vine
207 High Street
Waltham Cross
Hertfordshire EN8 7EB
Tel: 0992 651122

BMA Services Ltd
BMA House
Tavistock Square
London WC1H 9JP
Tel: 0800 181099

Coopers and Lybrand Deloitte
Plumtree Court
London EC1A 4HT
Tel: 071 583 5000
also at
Abacus Court, 6 Minshull Street
Manchester M1 3ED
Tel: 061 2369191

Ernst and Young
Becket House
Lambeth Palace Road
London SE1
Tel: 071 928 2000

The Royal Bank of Scotland PLC
Commercial Banking Services
PO Box 31
42 St Andrew Square
Edinburgh EH2 2YE
Tel: 031 523 5991

Touche Ross and Co
Columbia Centre
Market Street
Bracknell RG12 1PA
Tel: 0344 54445

Services and consultancy – legal

Alsop Wilkinson
6 Dowgate Hill
London EC4R 2SS
Tel: 071 248 4141

Barlow Lyde-Gilbert
Beaufort House
15 St Botolph Street
London EC3A 7NJ
Tel: 071 247 2277

Burton Copeland
Royal London House
196 Deansgate
Manchester M3 3NF
Tel: 061 834 7374

Cameron Markby Hewitt
Sceptre Court
40 Tower Hill
London EC3N 4BB
Tel: 071 702 2345

Capsticks
Upper Richmond Road
London SW15 2TT
Tel: 081 780 2211

Clyde and Co
51 Eastcheap
London EC3M 1JP
Tel: 071 623 1244

Crutes
7 Osborne Terrace
Newcastle upon Tyne NE2 1RQ
Tel: 091 291 5911

Field Fisher Waterhouse
Lincoln House
296–302 High Holborn
London WC1V 7JL
Tel: 071 831 9161

Ford and Warren
5 Park Square
Leeds LS1 2AX
Tel: 0532 436601

Hempsons
33 Henrietta Street
Covent Garden
London WC2E 8NH
Tel: 071 836 0011

Hill Dickinson Davis Campbell
Pearl Assurance House
Derby Square
Liverpool L2 9XL
Tel: 051 236 5400

Irwin Mitchell
St Peter's House
Hartshead
Sheffield S1 2EL
Tel: 0742 767777

J Tickle and Co
Victoria House
Vernon Place
London WC1B 4DP
Tel: 071 405 2391

Leathes Prior
74 The Close
Norwich NR1 4DR
Tel: 0603 610911

Le Brasseur and Monier-Williams
71 Lincoln's Inn Fields
London WC2A 3JF
Tel: 071 405 6195

Mackrell Turner Garrett
Inigo Place
31 Bedford Street
Strand
London WC2E 9EH
Tel: 071 240 0521

McKenna and Co
Mitre House
160 Aldersgate Street
London EC1A 4DD
Tel: 071 606 9000

Mills and Reeves
3–7 Rockwell Street
Norwich NR2 4TJ
also at
Francis House
112 Hills Road
Cambridge CB2 1PH

Morgan Bruce
Bradley Court, Park Place
Cardiff CF1 3DP
Tel: 0222 233677

Nabarro Nathanson
50 Stratton Street
London W1X 5FL
Tel: 071 493 9933

Pannone March Pearson
123 Deansgate
Manchester M3 2BU
Tel: 061 832 3000

Rakisons
27 Chancery Lane
London WC2A 1NF
Tel: 071 404 5212

Reynolds Porter Chamberlain
Chichester House
278–282 High Holborn
London WC1V 7HA
Tel: 0711 242 2877

Simpson Curtis
41 Park Square
Leeds LS1 2NS
Tel: 0532 433433

Taylor Joynson Garrett
180 Fleet Street
London EC4A 2NT
Tel: 071 430 1122

Wansbrough
103 Temple Street
Bristol BS99 7UD
Tel: 0272 268981

Services and consultancy – management, marketing and PR

Dunedin Management Consulting Ltd
39 Palmerston Place
Edinburgh EH12 5AU
Tel: 031 226 3148

Llewelyn-Davies Weekes
Brook House
2–16 Torrington Place
London WC1E 7HN
Tel: 071 637 0181

The London Health-Care Information Centre
Aviation Hosue
129 Kingsway
London WC2B 6NH
Tel: 071 831 8771

LSJ Healthcare
162 High Street
Newmarket
Suffolk CB8 9AQ
Tel: 0638 666272

McGilvery PR and Marketing
67 Lawnside
Blackheath
London SE3 9HL
Tel: 081 852 9350

Medi-Link International
Hennerton Farm
Wargrave
Berkshire RG10 8LT
Tel: 071 224 9091

Paramedex International Ltd
15 St Mary's Street
Lincoln LN5 7EQ
Tel: 0522 544515

Percy Thomas Partnership
20 Victoria Street
Nottingham NG1 2EX
Tel: 0602 587095

Royal National Orthopaedic Hospital Trust
Brockley Hill
Stanmore
Middlesex HA7 4LP
Tel: 081 954 2300

Services and consultancy – pharmaceutical selling

Zafash MTD Ltd
233 Old Brompton Road
London SW5 0EA
Tel: 071 373 3506

Services and consultancy – training and recruitment

David Lewis Centre
Mill Lane
Warford
Near Alderley Edge
Cheshire SK9 7UD
Tel: 0565 872613

Llewelyn-Davies Weeks
Brook House
2–16 Torrington Place
London WC1E 7HN
Tel: 071 637 0181

NHS Training Directorate
Hospital Estate Management and
Training Centre
Eastwood Park
Falfield, Wotton under Edge
Gloucestershire GL12 8DA
Tel: 0454 260207

Paramedex International Ltd
15 St Mary's Street
Lincoln LN5 7EQ
Tel: 0522 544515

Practice Personnel
12 Clousden Grange
Forest Hall
Newcastle upon Tyne NE12 0YW
Tel: 091 268 2172

Reynolds Training Services Ltd
Unit 6, Fleece Yard
Printers Mews
Buckinghamshire MK18 1JX
Tel: 0280 822728

Riverside Health Authority
Thomas Macauley Ward
Westminster Hospital
Dean Ryle Street
London SW1P 2AP
Tel: 081 746 8234

Stop Smoking
PO Box 100
Plymouth
Devon PL1 1RG
Tel: 0752 709506

The Training Department
104–108 Oxford Street
London W1N 9FA
Tel: 071 580 6312

Services and consultancy – travel health

British Airways Travel Clinics
7 Bury Place
London WC1A 2LA
Tel: 071 831 3266

Hospital For Tropical Diseases Travel Clinic
1 Queens House
1st Floor
180–182 Tottenham Court Road
London W1P 9LE
Tel: 071 637 9899

Liverpool School of Tropical Medicine
Pembroke Street
Liverpool L3 5QA
Tel: 051 708 9393

London School of Tropical Medicine
Keppel Street
London WC1
Tel: 071 636 8636
operates
Medical Advice Service for Travellers Abroad (MASTA)
Tel: 071 631 4408

Services and consultancy – video services

CTVC
Hillside Studios
Merry Hill Road
Bushey
Hertfordshire WD1 2DR
Tel: 081 950 1437

Viewtech Film and Video
161 Winchester Road
Brislington
Bristol BS4 3NJ
Tel: 0272 773422

Skin clinic – tattoo removal

Clearway Clinic Plc
Head Office
41–43 Derngate
Northampton NN1 1UE
Tel: 0604 602684

Specialist patient care/treatment

The Endocrine Centre
69 Wimpole Street
London W1M 7DE
Tel: 071 935 2440

Waste management

J G Industrial Products
28 Cabragh Road
Grange, Armagh
Northern Ireland
Tel: 0861 522573

Medical Waste International Ltd
Blue Circle House
Holborough
Snodland
Kent ME6 4PH
Tel: 0634 244138

Neatworld Ltd
7–9 Tottenham Lane
Crouch End
London N8 9DN
Tel: 081 341 9556

Royal National Orthopaedic Hospital Trust
Brockley Hill
Stanmore
Middlesex HA7 4LP
Tel: 081 954 2300

Surrey-Sac Products Ltd
Trinity Road
Richmond
Surrey TW9 2LG
Tel: 081 948 8822

Useful Addresses

Age Concern
Astral House, 1268 London Road
London SW16 4EJ
Tel: 081 679 8000

Action on Smoking & Health (ASH)
109 Gloucester Place
London W1H 3PH
Tel: 071 935 3519

Association of Medical Secretaries, Practice Administrators and Receptionists
Tavistock House North
Tavistock Square
London WC1H 9LN
Tel: 071 387 6005

Barnado's
Tanners Lane
Barkingside, Ilford
Essex IG6 1QG
Tel: 081 550 8822

British Diabetic Association
10 Queen Anne Street
London W1M 0BD
Tel: 071 323 1531

British Dietetic Association
7th Floor, Elizabeth House
22 Suffolk Street
Queensway
Birmingham B1 1LS
Tel: 021 643 5483

British Medical Association
BMA House, Tavistock Square
London WC1H 9JP
Tel: 071 387 4499

BMA Local Offices
East Anglia: 0223 64539
Edinburgh: 031 662 4820
Glasgow: 041 332 1862
Mersey: 051 709 5660
Northern: 091 261 7131
Northern Ireland: 0232 663272
North Thames: 071 388 8296
North Western: 061 434 9231
Oxford: 0865 59621
South Thames: 081 660 5558
South Western: 0272 227645
Trent: 0742 721705
Wales: 0222 485336
Wessex: 0962 856760
West Midlands: 021 456 1402
Yorkshire: 0532 458745

Cancer Relief Macmillan Fund
Anchor House
15–19 Britten Street
London SW3 3TZ
Tel: 071 351 7811

Charity Commission
St Albans House
57–60 Haymarket
London SW1Y 4QH
Tel: 071 210 3000

Chartered Society of Physiotherapy
14 Bedford Row
London WC1R 4ED
Tel: 071 242 1941

College of Health
St Margaret's House
Old Ford Road
London E2 9PL
Tel: 081 983 1225

Department of Health
Richmond House
79 Whitehall
London SW1A 2NS
Tel: 071 210 3000

Northern Ireland:
Dundonald House
Upper Newtonards Road
Belfast BT4 3SB
Tel: 0232 520000

Family Planning Association
27–35 Mortimer Street
London W1N 7RJ
Tel: 071 631 0555

General Medical Council
44 Hallam Street
London W1N 6AE
Tel: 071 580 7642

General Optical Council
41 Harley Street
London W1N 2DJ
Tel: 071 580 3898

General Practice Finance Corporation
Tavistock House North
Tavistock Square
London WC1H 9JL
Tel: 071 387 5274

Haemophilia Society
123 Westminster Bridge Road
London SE1 7HR
Tel: 071 928 2020

Health and Safety Executive
Baynards House, 1 Chepstow Place
Westbourne Grove
London W2 4TF
Tel: 071 243 6630

Health Visitors' Association
50 Southwark Street
London SE1 1UN
Tel: 071 378 7255

Her Majesty's Stationery Office Publications Centre
PO Box 276
London SW8 5DT
Tel: 071 873 0011

Independent Doctors Forum
Broadgate Medical Centre
Exchange Arcade
175 Bishopsgate
London EC2M 3WA
Tel: 071 972 9972

Independent Healthcare Association
22 Little Russell Street
London WC1A 2NT
Tel: 071 430 0537

Institute of Health Services Management
75 Portland Place
London W1N 4AN
Tel: 071 580 5041

Kings Fund Centre
126 Albert Street
London NW1 7NF
Tel: 071 267 6111

Medical and Dental Defence Union of Scotland Ltd
120 Blythwood Street
Glasgow G2 4EH
Tel: 041 221 3663

The Medical Defence Union Ltd
3 Devonshire Place
London W1N 2EA
Tel: 071 486 6181

Medical Practices Committee, England and Wales
Room 110
Eileen House
80–94 Newington Causeway
London SE1 6EF
Tel: 071 972 2930

Medical Practices Committee, Scotland
Room A023
Trinity Park House
South Trinity Road
Edinburgh EH5 3PY
Tel: 031 552 6255

The Medical Protection Society Ltd
50 Hallam Street
London W1N 6DE
Tel: 071 637 0541

Medical Women's Federation
Tavistock House North
Tavistock Square
London WC1H 9HX
Tel: 071 387 7765

Medico-Legal Society
Barlow Lyde-Gilbert
Beaufort House
15 St Botolph's Street
London EC3A 7NJ
Tel: 071 247 2277

MENCAP
Mencap National Centre
123 Golden Lane
London EC1Y 0RT
Tel: 071 454 0454

MIND
22 Harley Street
London W1N 2ED
Tel: 071 637 0741

National Blood Authority (NBA)
Oak House
Reeds Crescent
Watford
Hertfordshire WD1 1QH
Tel: 0923 212121

National Care Homes Association
5 Bloomsbury Place
London WC1A 2HA
Tel: 071 436 1871

National Childbirth Trust
Alexander House
Oldham Terrace
London W3 6NH
Tel: 081 992 8637

National Schizophrenia Fellowship
28 Castle Street
Kingston upon Thames
Surrey KT1 1SS
Tel: 081 547 3937

NSPCC
67 Saffron Hill
London EC1N 8RS
Tel: 071 242 1626

Prescription Pricing Authority
Bridge House
152 Pilgrim Street
Newcastle upon Tyne NE1 6SN
Tel: 091 232 5371

Registered Nursing Home Association Ltd
Calthorpe House
Hagley Road
Edgbaston B16 8QY
Tel: 021 454 2511

RoSPA
Cannon House, The Priory
Queensway
Birmingham B4 6BS
Tel: 021 200 2461

The Royal College of General Practitioners
14 Princes Gate
London SW7 1PU
Tel: 071 581 3232

Royal College of Midwives
15 Mansfield Street
London W1M 0BE
Tel: 071 580 6523

Royal College of Nursing
20 Cavendish Square
London W1M 0AB
Tel: 071 409 3333

Royal College of Obstetrics and Gynaecology
27 Sussex Place, Regent's Park
London NW1 4RG
Tel: 071 262 5425/402 2317

Royal College of Physicians
11 St Andrews Place
London NW1 4LE
Tel: 071 935 1174

Royal College of Surgeons
Lincoln's Inn Fields
London WC2A 3PN
Tel: 071 405 3474

Royal Society of Medicine
1 Wimpole Street
London W1M 8AE
Tel: 071 408 2119

Society of Chiropodists
53 Welbeck Street
London W1M 7HE
Tel: 071 486 3381

Society of Occupational Medicine
6 St Andrews Place
London NW1 4LB
Tel: 071 486 2641

St Johns Ambulance
1 Grosvenor Crescent
London SW1X 7EF
Tel: 071 235 5231

Index of Advertisers

Benson & Co 95
The Bethlem Royal Hospital and Maudsley Hospital 25
The British College of Acupuncture 41
Biolab 169
Clearway Clinics 41
The David Lewis Centre 133
De Puy Healthcare 32–3
The Endocrine Centre 16
EMIS 85
General Healthcare (BMI) 58–9
The Hospital for Tropical Diseases Travel Clinic 10
Janssen Pharmaceutical Ltd *inside front cover*, 127
The London Clinic 62
The Manor House Hospital 116
The Medical Protection Society 8
Medi-Lab Ltd 171
NPS Health Option Scheme 35
Owen Mumford 71
Pharmax Ltd 150–52
Private Patients Unit Bloomsbury and Islington Health Authority 2
The Proudfoot School of Hypnosis and Psychotherapy 41
Queen Square Imaging Centre 148
Response Marketing (Nationwide) Ltd 41
The Royal Bank of Scotland 82
Royal National Orthopaedic Hospital Trust 138–9
School of Phytotherapy 177
Sheffield Pathology Services 71
Stop Smoking 95

Touche Ross and Company 111
Weightwatchers UK Ltd 118–19
The Yorkshire Clinic 95